"What are you willing to do that others will not, so your body can perform when theirs cannot?"

Library of Congress Cataloging-in-Publication Data is on file with the publisher.

ISBN: 978-0-9845721-3-7 Paperback

Find Dr. Rob Kominiarek online:

Dr. Rob's Medical Offices: **http://www.alphamaleinstitute.com/**

Dr. Rob in the Media: **http://www.americasfitnessdoctor.com**

More information on The Low T Book at **http://www.lowtbook.com**

Editing, graphics, digitalization and cover design by Greg Gallivan. Find Greg online at **http://www.switchphase.com/**

First Edition Printed July 2014.

ACKNOWLEGDEMENTS

I would like to take a moment and thank all the people who helped to create this book. Dave Braughler and his team from Greyden Press, I always have fun working with you to create the next piece in the puzzle. Greg Gallivan and his team, your constant efforts to help us bring this project to reality were invaluable. To my family, friends and patients who have held me to the highest standards of medical excellence, dedication, and the constant seeking of truth; your support fuels my drive.

TABLE OF CONTENTS

INTRODUCTION
FOREWORD

THE LOW T BOOK

A Man's 30 Day Guide to Improve Your Strength, Energy, Libido and Fitness

By: Robert A. Kominiarek D.O, FACOFP

There is no book, including this one that can ever replace the services of a qualified health care professional. Please discuss any and all subject matter in this book with your physician, so you can find your best path toward a healthy active life.

This book is written as a source of information only. The information contained in this book should by no means be considered a substitute for the advice of a qualified medical professional who should always be consulted before beginning any new exercise, diet, or health program.

All efforts have been made to ensure the accuracy of the information contained in the book as of the date published. The author and the publisher expressly disclaim responsibility for any adverse effects arising from the use or application of the information contained herein.

FOREWORD

In *The Low T Book*, Dr. Rob Kominiarek has made a clear, comprehensive and compelling case for the importance of the hormone testosterone in achieving and maintaining your health. As a fellow clinician who shares his conviction that age does ***not*** have to be synonymous with deteriorating health, I was especially pleased with Rob's request to write this foreword.

As Dr. Rob makes clear, a major component of healthy aging involves the body's hormones. These invisible messengers control every aspect of the body: weight gain, sleeping, breathing, muscle strength, brain function - you name it. As an endocrinologist who has spent over two decades studying the role of hormones in health and aging, I enthusiastically support Dr. Rob's refusal to accept that aging means a downward slide toward diseases such as diabetes, heart disease and osteoporosis. My own clinical practice and research in the emerging field of Precision Medicine - the personalization of health care - heartily supports Dr. Rob's thesis: testosterone is a major player when it comes to the revitalization of an individual's health.

The male patients that Dr. Rob and I advise are largely unaware of what goes on in their bodies internally, though they share one or more frustrating, hard-to-shake symptoms. These can include weight gain around the trunk, fatigue, loss of energy, anxiety, sleep disorders, difficulty recovering after exercise, sexual dysfunction, and lack of libido. In short, these are the "complaints of aging" and many men do not realize that these are indicators of *andropause*, the male equivalent to menopause. We know that testosterone plays a key role in many processes, such as retaining lean muscle, exercise recovery, sugar metabolism, and sexual function, to name several. We also know that the ailments of aging are integrally connected to the gradual drop in testosterone levels that begins in early adulthood. And we now know that testosterone can be harnessed to achieve peak physiological health as we age. Hormonal optimization along with quality sleep, nutrition, exercise, and effective stress management - proactively and simultaneously set in place - can alter your health trajectory.

Scientific data suggests it is possible to focus on interventions to improve the quality of your life and circumvent disorders of aging. Our clinical and pilot research studies support that the outcome will allow your **health** span to last for your **life** span. *The Low T Book* lays the facts out for you. It educates, enlightens, and has the potential to set you on the path to substantial renewal and recovery.

On a snowy day this past winter, Dr. Rob traveled into Manhattan for a television appearance and made time to visit my office. We spent several hours deeply engrossed in discussion about medicine's exciting future, in which the rapidly advancing field of Precision Medicine, and the advent of genomics and epigenetics, will ultimately allow doctors to treat each patient as the unique individual he or she is. From that meeting and our subsequent discussions, I have every indication to believe that Dr. Rob is squarely in the forefront of that future.

By Florence Comite MD
September 8, 2014

Dr. Comite is a graduate of Yale School of Medicine where she taught for 25 years, as an Associate Clinical Professor. She is the author of the Amazon best-seller book for men: **Keep It Up: The Power of Precision Medicine to Conquer Low T and Revitalize Your Life**, *published by Rodale. Florence Comite MD currently has a private practice in Manhattan, where she manages the health of individuals from all over the world.*

Chapter 1

The State of Male Health – What You Don't Know May Kill You

Every Man's Problem!

In men the symptoms of testosterone deficiency are often under diagnosed and undertreated. Many a man intuitively feels the change in his health only to inquire about his testosterone level and be told that, "it's fine" when in reality it is horribly deficient. Based on total testosterone concentration, the prevalence of hypogonadism in men reporting to primary care offices is estimated to be 38.7%. The FDA estimates that somewhere between 4 and 5 million men suffer from low testosterone with less than 5% of men ever being tested.

The medical conditions that are significantly associated among hypogonadal men included increase in abdominal fat, hypertension, hyperlipidemia, diabetes, metabolic syndrome, hypertension, heart attack, stroke, and cancer. As men age, they are susceptible to conditions that share many of the same symptoms similar to hypogonadism. The presence of these conditions may even mask underlying hypogonadism and negatively impact quality of life.

After age 20 male hormones begin a slow gradual decline, some falling about 14% every decade. By the time a man reaches 40, he's lost almost half the necessary hormones he had at 20 years old. But you don't have to be middle-aged or older to experience hormone deficiency. Hormone deficiencies are strongly associated with the onset of these serious diseases that often lead to disabling conditions:

- Cardiovascular disease
- Strokes
- Diabetes
- Dementia
- Osteoporosis
- Depression
- Vascular dysfunction
- Metabolic Syndrome
- Cancer

There are striking similarities among the many men who have sought my assistance with what they thought was just low testosterone. More often than not their initial biomarkers disclose significant health risks besides low testosterone. These medical threats to their health usually include cholesterol derangement, pre-diabetes, elevated Hemoglobin A1c, elevated homocysteine; which is a biomarker for inflammation, suboptimal Vitamin D, magnesium, zinc, sarcopenia (muscle wasting), cardiovascular deconditioning, osteopenia, endothelial dysfunction, growth hormone deficiency, hypothyroidism and more. Having low levels of vitamin D along with low levels of testosterone raises a man's risk from all-cause mortality significantly.

There are three disease states that have become all too commonplace over the last decade. These are diabetes, cardiovascular disease, and metabolic syndrome, all of which are associated with low testosterone. In chapter four I will discuss why it is more about your heart above all else, because what difference does it make if you fix your T, but don't care for your heart?

Diabetes and low testosterone

Diabetes in America affects some 27 million people and it is estimated that around 67 million people have pre-diabetes, both of which have a strong association with low testosterone. Numerous studies have demonstrated the serious effects of consistently elevated HgbA1c levels seen in diabetes on the oxidation of LDL cholesterol. Epidemiologic studies have shown that *higher levels* are associated with *substantially higher risks* for:

- Congestive Heart Failure
- Heart Disease
- Heart Attacks
- Strokes
- Brain Atrophy
- Cancer
- Vascular Endothelial Dysfunction
- Increased Blood Clotting
- High Blood Pressure
- Diabetes
- Thyroid disorders

It is strongly recommended to identify and treat impaired fasting glucose early as its progression into diabetes and coronary artery disease is silent and progressive until a catastrophic event occurs. This is one of the many reasons why a comprehensive plan to improve your health that encompasses healthy nutrition, exercise, lifestyle adjustments and hormone restoration when necessary is critical to your male health.

Metabolic Syndrome and low testosterone

Metabolic syndrome which is becoming all too common among American men, describes a cluster of conditions that typically includes the presence of 3 or more of the following: elevated blood pressure or hypertension, elevated waist circumference which is central obesity or "belly fat", elevated fasting glucose which is a measure of insulin resistance, elevated triglycerides (hypertriglyceridemia), and reduced levels of "good" HDL cholesterol, all often seen in men with low testosterone.

Metabolic syndrome is associated with increased risk of developing more serious chronic illnesses, such as cardiovascular disease and type 2 Diabetes. In addition to elevated blood pressure and triglycerides, several other risk factors for heart disease may also be present with metabolic syndrome, including elevated levels of "bad" LDL cholesterol (hypercholesterolemia) and an altered body composition, which is an unfavorable ratio of unhealthy fat to healthier lean body tissues, such as muscle.

Here are some alarming statistics as it stands today:

- As many as 1 in 3 American adult men have insulin resistance, even though most don't know it.
- About 1 in 3 U.S. adult men has high blood pressure.
- Over 1 in 3 American adult men is overweight or obese, placing them at greater risk for metabolic syndrome, heart disease, and low testosterone.
- 1 in 3 U.S. adult men may have metabolic syndrome, the likelihood of which increases with age
- More than 1 in 3 American adult men have one or more forms of cardiovascular disease.

Alarmingly, almost 50% of adult Americans suffer from at least one of these chronic illnesses and for adults over 65 years of age, more than 50% are being treated for multiple chronic conditions. Proactively treating low testosterone to prevent any and all of the chronic medical conditions such as cardiovascular disease, vascular dysfunction and osteoporosis can preserve and maintain a high quality of life for decades to come and spare the individual heartache and misery.

The CDC estimated that the cost for managing these chronic illnesses in the United States accounts for close to 78 percent of our health care expenditures. Having one of these chronic illnesses will mean that you will most likely spend 3 times as much as a man without any chronic disease, making prevention our and your number one goal.

Besides what we spend there is also what we lose. Having one of these chronic diseases with low testosterone leads to decreased productivity and absenteeism from work. The CDC estimated that almost 7 out of 10 deaths are due to chronic disease from heart attacks, strokes, and cancer, which all have a connection to low testosterone in both men and women. Chronic illness caused in part by low testosterone steals years of life from our potential health and vitality. The burden of discomfort, pain, and progressive dysfunction and disability that an individual suffers cannot be truly measured. As men, we see ourselves as providers and protectors of our family, friends, and nation and to become a burden to the ones we love and the pain and anguish of surrendering the quality of our lives is unimaginable.

The only cure for hormonal deficiency is restoration of hormone balance!

Many of the symptoms of male hormone imbalances come on very gradually. You may not notice them at first, but as more symptoms appear and become worse over time, they rob you of your youth and vitality. These symptoms may include:

- Erectile dysfunction
- Low libido
- Decreased bone mass or osteoporosis
- Night sweats or hot flashes
- Decrease in energy or "get up and go"
- Decline in neuromuscular response

- Depression or anxiety
- Decreased sense of well being
- Constipation or increased bowel movements
- Increased body fat & male breasts
- Hair loss
- Fatigue or lack of energy
- Memory loss
- Decline in focus or concentration
- Heart palpitations
- Sleep apnea or insomnia
- Mood swings or irritability
- Muscle loss or weakness

Many times people often mistake the symptoms of testosterone deficiency in men with signs of aging. The good news is that these hormone imbalances are easily correctible, when you take action.

Most men measure their health by the triad of manliness. What they do for a living, how many dollars are in their bank account, and what's their status between the sheets! If anyone of these areas is not in alignment then all is wrong with the world. But, what most men forget to take into account is that their personal health is really the cornerstone to their overall well-being. When their health suffers so does every other aspect of their life.

Alarmingly, the level of testosterone in men has been steadily declining over the past 2 decades. The reasons for this decline are not completely clear. A study has suggested that neither aging nor changes in certain health factors, such as obesity, smoking, or metabolic disease can completely explain the phenomenon.

According to Thomas G. Travison, Ph.D., of the New England Research Institutes (NERI) in Watertown, Mass., and lead author of the study: *Male serum testosterone levels appear to vary by generation, even after age is taken into account*:

"In 1988, men who were 50 years old had higher serum testosterone concentrations than did comparable 50-year-old men in 1996. This suggests that some factors other than age may be contributing to the observed declines in testosterone over time."

Personally over the last decade I have noticed a drastic increase in the number of younger men with testosterone deficiency linked to sometimes-identifiable lifestyle and environmental causes. Later in the book I will discuss natural remedies to increase testosterone levels that have been lowered by these alarming environmental trends.

It is my opinion that the constant low level exposure to the abundance of chemicals with estrogen like activity that permeate the majority of plastics, food wrappers, household chemicals, pharmaceuticals, pesticides, thermal paper, and food items play an ever increasing role in decreasing testosterone levels. So what can you do to limit your exposure to chemicals with estrogen like activity?

- Eat Organic
- Use Natural Cleaning Products
- Use Natural Personal Care Products
- Avoid scented or fragrant oils

Testosterone is the primary male sex hormone. It is important for maintaining bone and muscle mass throughout life. Insufficient levels of testosterone have been linked to diabetes, low libido, and other medical conditions. Typically, testosterone levels in men peak around their late 20s, and then begin a gradual decline from age 30 onward. Testosterone also is present in women, but at significantly lower levels.

Travison and colleagues based their study on data from the Massachusetts Male Aging Study (MMAS). The MMAS comprised three separate data-collection periods over 17 years (1987-89, 1995-97, and 2002-04). The study involved collecting blood samples, as well as health and biographical data, from approximately 1,500 randomly selected men residing in the greater Boston area.

During each phase of the study, the researchers analyzed the subjects' blood samples to measure total testosterone, from which they also calculated the amount of "bioavailable testosterone". Bioavailable testosterone includes both free testosterone, which is unbound to proteins like albumin, and testosterone weakly bound to proteins like albumin. Bioavailable testosterone is available to tissues to support various functions within the body, because it is loosely bound.

The NERI team analyzed the data to compare men of similar ages during each phase of the study. After accounting for age and additional factors such as obesity, smoking, and medications, the researchers found that, each year, the subjects' total testosterone decreased an average of 1.2 and bio-available testosterone decreased an average of 1.3 percent.

For men 65-69 years of age in this study, average total testosterone levels fell from 503 ng/dL in 1988 to 423 ng/dL in 2003. A normal, asymptomatic, healthy adult male usually has blood total testosterone concentrations that range anywhere from 300-1000 ng/dL. In my experience that number is generally in excess of 550 ng/dL.

Travison acknowledged that hormone concentrations in the blood are difficult to measure, primarily due to normal daily fluctuations. To ensure these changes did not bias the results, two samples were obtained at each visit, and all were taken early in the morning, when testosterone levels are at their highest.

In addition, each MMAS data collection period utilized the same laboratory and the same technology to analyze subjects' blood. "Nevertheless," said Travison, "time and technology march on, so it's impossible to completely rule out the influence of subtle changes in the way the samples were obtained or processed. That being said, our results appear to be consistent across the various waves of the study."

The researchers point out that, although subjects' current health was taken into account as part of the analysis, it is impossible to account for certain health or environmental influences that may have impacted the subjects' testosterone levels prior to being enrolled in the study.

"This analysis deals with men who were born between 1915 and 1945," said Travison, "but our baseline data were not obtained until the late 1980s, when the elder subjects were about 70 years old, and the youngest about 45. Events occurring in earlier decades could certainly help explain our results, if their effects persisted into recent years." It is also possible that current, but unmeasured, health or environmental factors could be the root cause of the observed declines.

A study by Dr. Araujo reported in the *Journal of Sexual Medicine* (Vol. 10, Issue 2, 2013) sought to quantify the cost burden imposed by testosterone deficiency in men.

After examining six national databases, scientists estimated that testosterone deficiency was affecting 13.4 percent of men between the ages of 45 and 74. They also estimated that testosterone deficiency is involved in the development of approximately 1.3 million new cases of cardiovascular diseases, 1.1 million new cases of diabetes, and more than 600,000 osteoporosis-related fractures in the first year it is present. Over a 20-year period, the researchers estimated that testosterone deficiency would be responsible for up to $525 billion in healthcare expenditures in the United States.

As this study points out, the cost of not treating testosterone deficiency is severe. Decreases in bone mass, muscle mass and strength, increases in metabolic syndrome, diabetes, cardiovascular disease, dementia, osteoporosis, and erectile dysfunction are all related to testosterone deficiency.

The most frequent complaint I hear from men with low testosterone is fatigue and lack of well-being. Other significant complaints include irritability, low libido, declining cognitive skills; concentration, memory, muscle loss, and weight gain around the mid-section. It comes as no surprise that:

"OPTIMUM HEALTH IS NO ACCIDENT. IT IS THE REWARD FOR TAKING A PREVENTATIVE AND PROACTIVE APPROACH TO YOUR PERSONAL HEALTH. HEALTHY NUTRITION, EXERCISE, AND PREVENTION ARE THE MOST POWERFUL PRESCRIPTION TO CORRECT HORMONE IMBALANCES. IN COMBINATION WITH HORMONE RESTORATION THERAPY WHEN NECESSARY, THEIR EFFECTS ARE IMPROVED QUALITY OF LIFE AND POTENTIAL LONGEVITY."

As such, every patient at our facility undergoes an intensive laboratory, diagnostic, and physical evaluation. Optimizing a man's testosterone level many times is a life changing treatment with numerous health, physical, and social benefits. I often hear from many of our clients, "I feel like me again!" And what could be better than feeling like you did when you were in your twenties? The optimization of the hypogonadal man's testosterone is a lifesaving treatment.

Chapter 2

Take Control of Your Man Health Now (What is Low T)

So where does this man juice come from exactly? Well testosterone is synthesized from cholesterol, which is an essential biochemical precursor for many hormones. It is the hormone responsible for normal growth, development and maintenance of male sex characteristics and its effects are body wide. It also directly affects lean body mass, strength, bone density, mood, cognitive skills, and sexual function. It is the primary androgenic and anabolic hormone in men and plays an important role in women as well.

Testosterone is produced by the testes in males and by the ovaries in females, with small amounts also produced by the adrenal glands in both men and women. Other hormones in an intricate and delicate dance of cascading hormones regulate the production and secretion of testosterone.

The hormonal and reproductive function of the testicles is regulated through interactions between the hypothalamus, the pituitary gland, and the gonads and is referred to as the Hypothalamic-Pituitary-Testicular Axis or H-P-T-A. The three glands communicate with each other through a cascade of hormones and a negative feedback loop to help maintain homeostatic levels. Altered cellular communication can disrupt this delicate balance.

Causes of Altered Cellular Communication:

- Stress
- Toxins
- Trauma
- Drugs
- Acute & Chronic Disease
- Lifestyle
- Nutrition
- Food Sensitivities
- Intracellular nutrient deficiencies

The release of gonadotropin-releasing hormone, GnRH, via the portal circulation from the hypothalamus to the pituitary stimulates the secretion of the two gonadotropin hormones called luteinizing hormone, LH, and follicle-stimulating hormone, called FSH from the anterior pituitary. Luteinizing hormone facilitates the production and secretion of testosterone from the leydig cells of the testes, while FSH stimulates the production of sperm.

Testosterone, like the gonadotropins is secreted in a pulsatile fashion, which occurs throughout the entirety of the day. About 5-7mg/day of testosterone is released. The normal range of total testosterone, depending on the laboratory of course is 348-1197 ng/dL. A total testosterone less than 550 ng/dL is considered low and less than 350 ng/dL is almost always associated with symptoms. More importantly however, is not the number, but how the man is feeling.

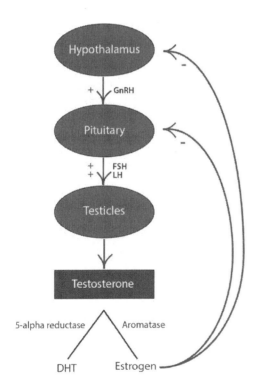

Testosterone is converted into two hormones called dihydrotestosterone or DHT and estrogen. The process by which testosterone is converted into estrogen by the aromatase enzyme is known as "aromatization".

Men with high body fat percentages, older men, and men taking certain medications, or males with a genetic predisposition to having higher than normal amounts of aromatase may experience higher conversion rates of testosterone into estrogen.

Estrogen is a very important hormone for men at the right concentration and estrogen plays an important role in bone, hair, heart, skin, and brain health as well as other functions in men. About 15%-20% of men will have issues with elevated estrogen levels while on testosterone therapy. Estrogen has some unwanted negative effects in that it down-regulates testosterone receptors and increases sex hormone binding globulin, which decreases the amount of bioavailable testosterone and diminishes the overall response. I will talk more about that later. Large amounts of estrogen can cause mood swings, enlarged breasts or gynecomastia, nipple tenderness, fat gain, water retention and the potential for a strong emotional need to eat chocolates while watch the "Notebook". I wish I could say I was kidding, but I have seen many a man become overly "sensitive" because of high estrogen levels.

The other metabolite of testosterone is dihydrotestosterone. DHT is a very potent androgen and is important for libido. In some men elevated DHT may cause male pattern baldness or benign prostatic hypertrophy. DHT has a positive effect on sexual desire but high levels of 5α-DHT increase the chance of hair loss, acne, oily skin and potential prostate issues.

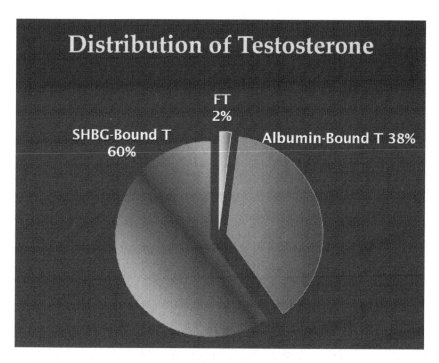

The majority of testosterone circulates in the blood bound to a carrier protein, which is a hormone produced in one area of the body and has its effect on another area it also assists the hormone to travel through the bloodstream. This carrier protein is called "sex hormone binding globulin," or SHBG. SHBG binds approximately 60% of testosterone. When testosterone is being carried by SHBG, it is considered "bound". Bound testosterone does not play an active role in the body; only the unbound or "free" testosterone is able to enter the different cells of the body and exert its androgenic and anabolic effects. Anything that affects the function or the amount of SHBG, like increasing estrogen levels, can also affect the total circulating amount of active testosterone.

It is not unusual in men over the age of 40 to have a normally functioning Hypothalamic-Pituitary-Testicular Axis producing total testosterone levels above 700 ng/dL with a low free testosterone level of say 24ng/dL., the normal range for Free T is 40-250 ng/dL., and because the liver is producing a large amount of SHBG, they have a high level say at 94 nmol/L, they have very little free testosterone in the bloodstream available for use by the body's tissues and they feel the full effects of having low testosterone.

About 38% percent of the body's testosterone is attached to albumin. Testosterone is not as tightly bound to albumin as SHBG, but it is still bound nonetheless. Like SHBG-bound testosterone, albumin-bound testosterone is biologically inactive. However, unlike testosterone bound to SHBG, the bind between albumin and testosterone is weak and can be easily broken in order to increase free testosterone.

About 2 percent of the testosterone in the body is metabolically available. This "free testosterone" is not attached to either albumin or SHBG that would prevent it from interacting with its receptor. (See diagram on following page)

The normal range for Free T is 40-250 ng/dL. Again what is important is not the exact number but how the individual feels. It is possible for a man to have a low Free T say of 90 ng/dL and be asymptomatic and another fellow have a high Free T of 220 ng/dL and be miserable with low libido, weak erections, moodiness, and no energy. No two men are alike.

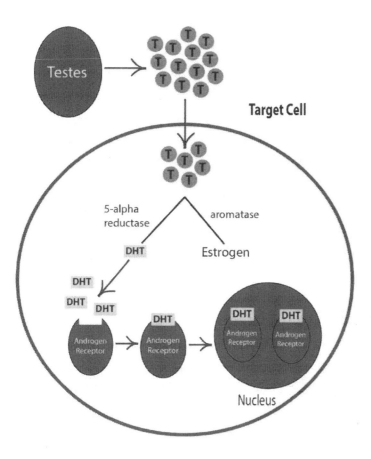

The diagram above shows the saturation of testosterone into the cell.

So what are symptoms of low testosterone?

- Can be more subtle than female menopause
- Progresses over 20 year period
- Starts in 30's
- A decline in muscle mass and strength
- Decrease of bone mass
- Increase in body fat, particularly abdominal and chest fat
- Metabolic Syndrome (coronary artery disease and increased cholesterol)
- Decline in cognitive skills, concentration and memory
- Decline in stamina and exertion performance

- Increased frequency of erectile dysfunction
- Decrease in sex drive and frequency of sexual thoughts
- Decreased sense of overall well-being
- Decreased perception of energy level and stamina
- Depression
- Fatigue
- Anxiety
- Aches and pains
- Loss of muscle elasticity

Decreased sex drive, erectile dysfunction, decreasing muscle mass, increasing body fat, less energy, decreased sense of well-being, fatigue and competition from younger men signals a declining virility. This decline could accompany the aging process, and be reluctantly accepted as fate. But, that does not need to be the case! However, I am also seeing an increase in younger men who experience these changes and this is not normal!

What is particularly disturbing is in the last 10 years the number of young men, under the age of 40, and some in their early 30's, that I see with hypogonadism associated with type 2 diabetes, obesity, high cholesterol, sexual dysfunction, toxin exposure, steroid abuse, and fatigue.

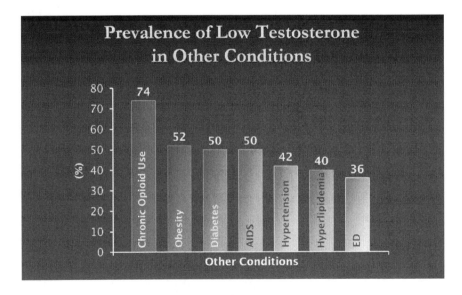

Men with testosterone deficiency are often under-diagnosed and often undertreated. The first signs of decline in testosterone are generally slightly vague: diminished subjective energy levels, increase in irritability, decline in mood, decline in cognitive performance, and loss of early morning erections.

Some men complain of infertility, decrease in beard and body hair, increase in body fat, decrease in muscle mass, gynecomastia (man boobs), increase in belly fat, changes in size or firmness of testicles.

While decreased sex drive and erectile quality are often the most frequent complaints associated with falling testosterone levels, they are actually some of the latest symptoms, with other symptoms present much sooner.

Often, men and their family members attribute these symptoms to psychosocial stressors or "aging" and do not seek medical help from their doctor. As testosterone declines, age-related drops in testosterone levels is associated with identifiable signs or symptoms: a decline in muscle mass and strength, decrease of bone mass, increase in body fat, particularly abdominal and chest fat, coronary artery disease, increasing cholesterol, decline in cognitive skills or concentration and memory, decline in stamina and exertion performance, increased frequency of erectile dysfunction, decline in sex drive and frequency of sexual thoughts, and decreased sense of overall well-being, decreased energy level and stamina.

Types of Hypogonadism and Andropause

Primary hypogonadism (hyper meaning high and hypo meaning low) also referred to as hypergonadotropic hypogonadism a condition where high levels levels of GnRH and LH are seen with low levels of testosterone. This occurs when the testicles fail to produce sufficient levels of testosterone for various reasons. This is also known as Andropause. Men in their fifties have usually begun to enter andropause and for some men this can occur even sooner.

Secondary hypogonadism results from hypothalamic or pituitary dysfunction resulting in hypogonadotropic hypogonadism and is characterized by disruption of central components of the H-P-T-A resulting in decreased levels of GnRH, LH, and FSH. In this type of hypogonadism, low levels of LH do not allow for the proper stimulation of the production of testosterone by the testes. This combination of low GnRH, low LH and low testosterone can be seen at any age and has multiple causes.

Primary Causes of Hypogonadism

- Congenital anorchidism
- Cryptorchidism (undescended testes)
- Mumps orchitis
- Sertoli-cell-only syndrome
- Noonan syndrome: phenotypic and genotypic males with physical signs of classic female Turner syndrome
- Radiation treatment/chemotherapy
- Testicular trauma/surgical procedures
- Autoimmune syndromes (anti-Leydig cell disorders)
- Genetic and developmental conditions: Klinefelter syndrome (1 in 1000 live births; most patients have 47, XXY genotype anomaly; however, mosaicism is also seen); androgen receptor and enzyme defects

Secondary causes of hypogonadism

- Pituitary macroadenoma
- Pituitary tumor, granulomas, abscesses
- Cranial trauma
- Radiation treatment
- Various medications
- Concussion
- Genetic conditions: Kallmann syndrome, Prader-Willi syndrome, Hyperprolactinemia

Mixed causes of hypogonadism

- Alcoholism
- Toxins
- Aging
- Chronic infections (human immunodeficiency virus)
- Corticosteroid treatment
- Hemochromatosis
- Systemic disease (liver failure, chronic kidney disease, sickle-cell disease)
- Substance Abuse

ADAM Questionnaire
Androgen Deficiency in the Aging Male (ADAM) Questionnaire

1. Do you have a decrease in sex drive?
2. Do you have a lack of energy?
3. Do you have a decrease in strength and/or endurance?
4. Have you lost height?
5. Have you noticed a decreased enjoyment in life?
6. Are you sad and/or grumpy?
7. Are your erections not as strong?
8. Has it been more difficult to maintain your erection throughout sexual intercourse?
9. Are you falling asleep after dinner?
10. Has your work performance deteriorated recently?

If you answered yes to number 1 or 7 or if you answered yes to more than 3 questions, you may have low testosterone.

In order to assess your current health status, you need to gather your biomarkers, and much more must be assessed that just the levels of total and free testosterone. Knowing your current baseline health profile will help to not only guide your therapy but help create an overall health and wellness plan that encompasses lifestyle, nutrition, exercise, and hormone therapy.

Appropriate lab work is crucial in diagnosing the potential different types and causes of hypogonadism and looking for any potential issues that may arise while on therapy. Below is a list of the initial screening labs that should be ordered in a fasting state.

Initial Screening Labs:

Total Testosterone	CBC
Testosterone Bioavailable or Weekly Bound	Insulin Immunoassay
	Lipid Panel or Lipoprotein panel
Testosterone Free	Prolactin
Cortisol AM	Vitamin D
SHBG	Cardiac CRP
HgA1c	Homocysteine
Thyroid Panel (TSH, FT4, FT3, rT3)	Iron
LH/FSH	TIBC
DHT	Ferritin
DHEA-Sulfate	IGF-1
Sensitive Estradiol	IGF-BP3
Liver panel	PSA
Serum Chemistries	Lyme titer if relevant by history
	Uric Acid
	Urinalysis

Strongly Consider These Labs:

IgG Food Sensitivity Testing
Micronutrient Testing
Lp-PLA2
MPO
NMR lipid, VAP, Berkley Heart Lab, or Cleveland Heart Lab
MTHFR
APO E

If you have a family history of an inherited blood clotting disorder or are not sure then you should consider these labs as well.

Factor V Leiden mutation
Factor VIII
Factor XI
Factor II (Prothrombin Gene)
Anticardiolipin antibody IgG/IgM
Lupus Anticoagulant

What labs to consider after the initiation of testosterone replacement therapy?

Follow up labs can be run at three to four weeks after starting therapy or changing the therapy dose or delivery method. This short amount of time provides for stabilization of the H-P-T-Axis, Sex Hormone Binding Globulin adjustment, and the pharmacodynamics of the testosterone delivery system. It takes time for the body to adjust to your chosen therapy delivery system.

Follow Up Labs:

Total Testosterone
Bioavailable Testosterone or "Free and Loosely Bound"
Free Testosterone if Bioavailable T is unavailable
Sensitive Estradiol
DHEA-S
FSH/LH
Hemoglobin and Hematocrit
Comprehensive Metabolic Panel
I would also recommend within the first 3 months of therapy to also test for the downstream metabolites of estrogen: 4-hydroxyestrone, 2-hydroxyestrone, 16-hydroxestrone, and the metabolites of testosterone, alpha DHT and beta DHT.

The hydroxylation of 2-hydroxyestrone (2-OH) and subsequent methylation to 2-methoxyestrone (2-MeO) produces the "beneficial" and balancing estrogens that every man needs for overall health especially for the positive cardiovascular, brain, and mood effects. These estrogens are eventually harmlessly excreted from the body. However, the hydroxylation of estrogens into 16 alpha hydroxyestrone (16α-OH) and its further reduction and binding to alpha and beta estrogen receptors can trigger the expression of target genes within the cell which may affect the health, function, and growth of estrogen responsive tissues in the uterus, breast, ovaries, cervix, bones, testicles, and prostate. This is where xenoestrogens like plasticizers, chemicals, drugs, and pesticides exert their harmful effects.

Even nastier is the hydroxylation of estrogen into 4-hydroxyestrone (4-OH) that is oxidized and is genotoxic and able to exert its potential carcinogenic effects upon the body's DNA. Desirable is the methylation of 4-hydroxyestrone (4-OH) into 4-methoxyestrone (4-MeO) with its eventual excretion from the body. The consumption of foods that contain and supplementation of vitamins A, C, E, α lipoic acid, lycopene, green tea, N-acetylcysteine for glutathione production, curcumin, selenium, carotenoids, and flavonoids help to reduce the potential oxidation of 4-hydroxyestrone into the unhealthy 3,4 Quinones.

Estrogen Metabolism

When it comes to estrogen metabolism, Estradiol (E2) is the more potent estrogen and along with Estrone (E1) and Estriol (E3) should be evaluated. Looking at the pathways from estrogen you can see that the desirable, protective pathway is to 2-OH-E1, the "good" estrogen. The pathways to 16-OH-E1, the "bad" estrogen, and 4-OH-E1, the "genotoxic", "carcinogenic" estrogen are not desirable. This is where healthful nutrition definitely comes into play in aiding the clearance of these harmful estrogens. There are also supplements that can assist here as well. The final step of estrogen metabolism is its methylation, which helps to protect the body against any potential harmful effects. The "hormone metabolite assessment" on the next page for this particular patient discloses that his hydroxylation of estrogen is in a healthful range, however phase 2 methylation activity is low and requires support and may be potentially linked to a genetic mutation.

This particular patient was homozygous for the MTHFR A1298C variant 2 SNPs (single nucleotide polymorphism) affecting his ability for appropriate phase 2 methylation of estrogens. Supporting his body's methylation ability would be advisable.

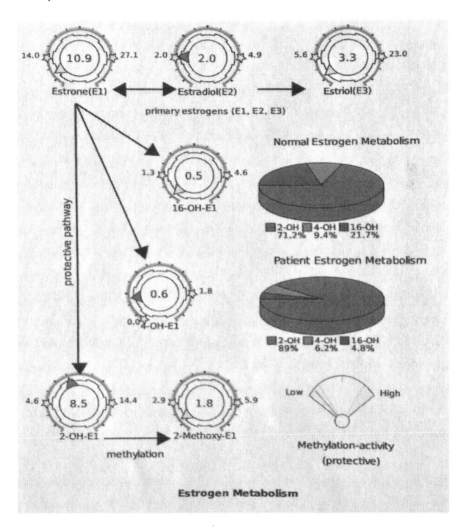

Estrogen Metabolism

MTHFR is extremely important in controlling the metabolism of the B vitamin known as folic acid. Folic acid is crucial to numerous functions of the brain, heart, blood, and immune system. The simple supplementation of 5-methyltetrahydrofolate from a nutritional supplement will decrease his risk for heart disease, dementia, depression, and improve his methylation.

As it turned out this man had high levels of homocysteine as well, in which 5-methyltetrahydrofolate supplementation would assist in lowering. Numerous studies have demonstrated the deleterious effects of high homocysteine levels. Epidemiologic studies have shown that *higher levels* are associated with *substantially higher risks* for:

- Congestive Heart Failure
- Heart Disease
- Heart Attacks
- Strokes
- Vascular Endothelial Dysfunction
- Increased Blood Clotting
- High Blood Pressure
- Diabetes
- Thyroid disorder

On my first rotation as a third year medical student many years ago a very wise internist said to me, *"The eye only sees what the mind knows."* I have never forgotten these powerful words and nothing could be truer when it comes to testosterone replacement therapy. We are only beginning to scratch the surface of this powerful therapy and we do not know what we don't know yet, which is why testosterone replacement therapy is not to be taken lightly.

Taking control of your man health is ultimately your responsibility. You are the Commander of your own health, it is up to you to work with your physician to understand and develop your personalized "plan of attack" to conquer and mitigate potential disease risk before it strikes. Gathering your personal biomarkers (labs and tests) for your physician is just like a commander in the military supplying his warriors with the necessary weapons and tools to get the job done in battle. The more ammunition and weapons you help your physician collect the more personalized your health care will become. Health care for men has taken a substantial move forward over the last decade thanks to the tireless work of numerous researchers and physicians we may never have the privilege of knowing, but to whom we certainly owe a debt of gratitude. Taking control of your man health and living a life full of vitality and free of disease honors their tireless efforts to improve our lives.

Low T Patient Profile: **Iron is for Lifting not Drinking!**

Doug, a 38 year old, athletic male with a 2-year history of declining endurance and athletic performance complaining of growing persistent fatigue, lethargy, altered sleep, decreased libido, and erectile quality. Also senses a decreased enjoyment in life and inability to make it through the day without feeling like he has to lie down. Patient states: "I feel like someone turned off my internal battery!"

DXA: Excellent bone mineralization, body composition 9.8% free fat mass
VO2: Fair results but feels "wiped out" after test, experienced palpitations at 158bpm
Neurocognitive evaluation: Decreased verbal memory and speed
Carotid Ultrasound with CIMT: No signs of plaque or thickening
VENDYS Testing: Excellent

Labs:

Liver panel: normal
CBC: normal
PSA: 0.7
Insulin: 9.0uIU/mL
Lipid Panel: normal
Prolactin:
Cortisol AM: 2.3!
LH: 7.0 mIU/mL!
Total Testosterone: 237ng/dL!
Free Testosterone: 6.2pg/mL!
Sensitive Estradiol: 12.6pg/mL

DHT: 56 ng/dL
SHBG: 26.8nmol/L
DHEA Sulfate: 168.9ug/dL !
Vitamin D: 24.2ng/mL!
Serum Iron: 300ug/dL!
Serum Ferritin: 195ng/mL
TSH: 4.0 uIU/mL!
fT3: 3.1 pg/mL
fT4: 1.09 ng/dL
Glucose: 79mg/dL
HgA1c: 5.0

Physical Examination revealed:

Obviously fatigued appearance, but well-nourished with excellent muscle structure
Low normal blood pressure 112/64, 110/62, 108/60
Mild thyroid swelling
Small testicles
DRE: unremarkable

Considerations for Differential Diagnosis:

Mixed Hypogonadism
Excessive Iron Intake vs. Hemochromatosis (an iron storage disease)
Subclinical Hypothyroidism
DHEA Deficiency
Vitamin D deficiency
Adrenal Fatigue
Parasympathetic Overtraining Syndrome (addisonoid)

Further investigation Reveals:

Drinks water exclusively from home well
Tests on well water reveal high iron level!

Therapy and Recommendations:

Don't drink your well water!
Heavy Metal Detoxification Program
Ergocalciferol 50,000 IU weekly x 4 then, Vitamin D 5000IU Sublingual QD
DHEA 25mg BID
Armour Thyroid 30mg Q AM
8 oz. warm water with Sea Salt upon rising in the AM
No Alcohol
No caffeine
Restorative Sleep in bed by 10PM
No training x 4 weeks, then return to training at 60% effort 3 days per week not to exceed a heart rate of 120bpm.

Subjective Patient Report

Feels drastic improvement inside 14-day period
No longer feels the need to lie down in afternoon
Anxious to workout

Follow Up Lab at 90 days:

Liver panel: normal
CBC: normal
Lipid Panel: normal
Prolactin:
Cortisol AM: 17.0
LH: 4.0 mIU/mL
Total Testosterone: 702ng/dL
Free Testosterone: 18.0pg/mL
Sensitive Estradiol: 16.6pg/mL

DHT: 58ng/dL
SHBG: 26.0nmol/L
DHEA Sulfate: 399.0ug/dL
Vitamin D: 60.2ng/mL
Serum Iron: 145ug/dL
Serum Ferritin: 195ng/mL
TSH: 1.0 uIU/mL
fT3: 2.1 pg/mL
fT4: 1.09 ng/dL

Take Home Point:

Investigate the cause of the hypogonadism and correct underlying deficiencies before committing yourself to a therapy that is not clinically needed... Just yet!

Chapter 3

Great Health Equals Great Sex

If you want more sex in your life then you have to put more life in your sex! And life starts with the foods you choose to eat and the amount of exercise you get. Research has demonstrated that the more exercise a person gets the less likely they will experience sexual dysfunction. Exercise boosts your body physically, emotionally, reduces stress, elevates mood, and increases confidence especially in the bedroom! Sex is a contact sport for sure and its physical requirements will rival that of any sport. In order to have great sex you have to have abundant energy, high aerobic capacity, strength, stamina, mobility, health and above all: blood flow.

"Because if the blood don't flow the sex is a no go"!

Keeping the blood flowing starts with your nutrition. The types of foods you eat, the vitamins and minerals you take, the amount of water you drink, and the adequate amounts of rest, the types of strenuous exercise you perform all help to create an internal environment that produces an abundance of sex hormones that stimulate sexual desire.

Inadequate amounts of the sex hormones, referred to as andropause in men and menopause in women can lead to decreased libido, fatigue, weight gain, loss of muscle mass, loss of strength, poor skin tone, increased cardiovascular issues, decreased bone density, disturbed sleep, and depression. Correcting these deficiencies all starts with proper nutrition and adequate exercise.

Having great sex all starts with being in excellent health and being in excellent health means no smoking, drinking limited amounts of alcohol, eating healthy balanced meals with appropriate amounts of healthy fat, exercising often, and drinking plenty of water.

Men, if you are not having at least 3-5 morning erections per week regardless of your age, go see your doctor. Lack of erections is a tell-tale sign of other health issues such as diabetes, vascular disease, and heart disease. Decreased libido and poor erectile quality are actually some of the later findings that there is a health problem.

To naturally increase your sex hormones do the following:

- Eat healthy meals daily
- Eat lean proteins like chicken, turkey, and lean beef
- Eat healthy fish with omega 3 fatty acids like salmon
- Eat plenty of green, leafy vegetables
- Eat low sugar fruits like berries and apples
- Avoid sugar
- Drink plenty of water
- Get adequate amounts of rest
- Do intense short exercises
- Limit unneeded stress
- Limit alcohol
- AND ABOVE ALL STOP SMOKING!

Keeping the blood flowing

What I am talking about here is having healthy endothelium. Endothelium is the thin interior lining of the blood vessel wall. The endothelium of the blood vessel forms the interface between the blood and your body. These endothelial cells secrete important substances such as *nitric oxide (NO)* which controls blood pressure, creates vascular tone, regulates chemical reactions, prevents oxidation and coagulation, and controls inflammatory processes. This thin lining can be damaged in different disease processes that all have one thing in common is inflammation. Inflammation is the silent killer that can start even in childhood only to later reveal itself during adulthood in damaged vessels, hypertension, erectile dysfunction, heart attacks, and strokes.

Here are the important vascular actions of nitric oxide:

- Direct vasodilation (flow dependent and receptor mediated)
- Indirect vasodilation by inhibiting vasoconstrictor influences (e.g., inhibits angiotensin II and sympathetic vasoconstriction)
- Anti-thrombotic effect - inhibits platelet adhesion to the vascular endothelium
- Anti-inflammatory effect - inhibits leukocyte adhesion to vascular endothelium; scavenges superoxide anion
- Anti-proliferative effect - inhibits smooth muscle hyperplasia

When nitric oxide production is impaired it results in:

- Vasoconstriction (e.g., coronary vasospasm, elevated systemic vascular resistance, hypertension)
- Thrombosis due to platelet aggregation and adhesion to vascular endothelium
- Inflammation due to upregulation of leukocyte and endothelial adhesion molecules
- Vascular hypertrophy and stenosis

Diseases or Conditions Associated with Abnormal Nitric Oxide Production

- High Blood Pressure
- Obesity
- High Cholesterol
- Diabetes
- Heart failure
- Atherosclerosis
- Accelerated Aging
- Cigarette smoking

Luckily, you have the power to change all this and create the internal environment to have healthy, fully functional endothelium by maintaining a healthy lifestyle of regular exercise, healthy nutrition, appropriate supplementation, drinking plenty of water and avoiding the endothelial damaging effects of smoking. Remember, if the blood don't flow the sex is a no go!

We can also directly test the vascular endothelium with a VENDYS® vascular function Test. VENDYS® (pronounced VEN-diss) is a noninvasive diagnostic device used to measure vascular reactivity for early detection of cardiovascular disease and monitoring response to therapy.

How does VENDYS® work?

The VENDYS® test begins with an automated blood pressure measurement, followed by cuff occlusion of the right arm. During the cuff occlusion (2 to 5 minutes), fingertip temperature in the right hand falls because of the absence of warm circulating blood. Once the cuff is released, blood flow rushes into the forearm and hand, causing a temperature rebound (TR) in the fingertip, which is directly proportional to the vascular reactivity.

Watch Dr. Rob demonstrate the VENDYS test **http://bit.ly/vendyltb**

Why get tested?

Because prevention is the best treatment! Cardiovascular disease develops over many years and if undetected can have life-threatening consequences. Initially it is a silent process, often called subclinical atherosclerosis. VENDYS® testing provides you with a quick and easy way of determining if you are heading down a road towards heart attack, stroke, and other cardiovascular diseases.

Vascular dysfunction is considered to be the earliest clinically detectable stage of subclinical atherosclerosis. Unlike atherosclerosis, vascular dysfunction is reversible (with proper treatment).

What is the endothelium?

The endothelium is the inner lining of blood vessels, allowing blood to flow smoothly within them and actively maintaining physiological condition. Normal vascular function protects blood vessels from formation of atherosclerosis, a cause of cardiovascular disease.

What is vascular dysfunction?

The pathological state known as vascular dysfunction is the earliest clinically detectable stage of cardiovascular disease (which includes heart attacks, stroke, Peripheral Arterial Disease and many other diseases).

ATHEROSCLEROSIS

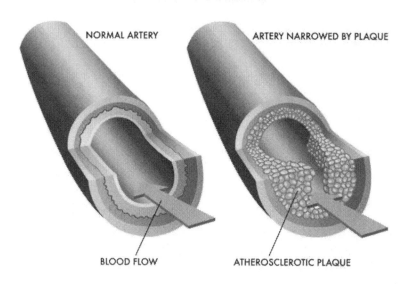

What will happen if it turns out that I have vascular dysfunction?

Your physician will evaluate the overall state of your health and discuss with you the most appropriate treatment options to improve your vascular function. These will usually include lifestyle modification measures (e.g. diet, food supplements, exercising), strict control of risk factors (e.g. quitting smoking), and supplement or prescription drug treatment. In some cases you will need to undergo more frequent monitoring and/or further testing of the cardiovascular system.

Remember - prevention is the best treatment!

Chapter 4

Your T is All About Your H (Heart)

It is well known that low testosterone and more specifically low free testosterone is associated with increased mortality from all causes in men. Men with normal levels of endogenous testosterone have significantly lower rates of cardiovascular mortality and from all causes and the survival time of men treated with testosterone versus men left untreated is longer as well.

There are no large prospective trials that have examined the association of cardiovascular disease and testosterone, but there are numerous observational studies that demonstrate the association between low T and cardiovascular disease. It is well known that testosterone therapy in the deficient male improves cardiovascular risk factors and there is no direct randomized controlled trial evidence that testosterone therapy is associated with increased cardiovascular risk.

So what is all the fuss about testosterone and heart attacks? That's because a couple of studies misrepresented their data. In the Finkle study, the pre-treatment rate for the first 90 days was 3.48 events per 1000 people and the post-treatment rate was 4.75 events per 1000 people for a difference of 1.27 events. This is not a significant difference and an absolutely uninformative study. Also, they never address the data set after 90 days wonder why? Possibly because it did not support their hypothesis.

Then there is the Vigen study, which contained major data errors and contamination of the data set that was not identified until after publication rendering the study not credible. This resulted in 29 medical societies and over 220 distinguished researchers and clinicians calling for JAMA to retract the study an issue an apology for printing "false information" that has "harmed public health, distorted medical science, and violated the trust between medical journals and the consumer" and referred to the printing of this article as "medical literature malpractice."

Despite these misguided studies, testosterone replacement therapy's beneficial effects are well documented as to the prevention of cardiovascular disease. The overwhelming majority of medical research does not demonstrate any relationship to increased risk of mortality, myocardial infarction or stroke. There are however numerous studies that do indicate the substantial benefits of TRT.

Testosterone replacement therapy in testosterone deficient, symptomatic patients improves:

- Sexual function and interest
- Bone mineral density
- Muscle Strength
- Increased exercise capacity
- Decreased hip to waist ratio
- Fat free mass
- Lean body mass
- Quality of erections (what we all really want anyways)
- Lipid profiles
- Insulin sensitivity
- Cardiac risk factors
- Mood stability
- Cognitive function
- Quality of Life
- Augments growth hormone secretion
- Increased time to ST segment depression during stress testing

Here are some additional issues with these studies:

- A retrospective cohort study of men with low testosterone levels who underwent coronary angiography and had low serum testosterone, categorized as initiating testosterone therapy if they filled a prescription for testosterone gel, patch, or injections following coronary angiography based on pharmacy-dispensing data. Once initiated, a patient was ASSUMED to have continued treatment until an outcome event occurred or the end of follow-up.

- There is no indication of appropriate follow up, monitoring of testosterone replacement therapy, or continuance of therapy among cohorts of this national retrospective study of men with low testosterone levels.

- Clinical trials have demonstrated that testosterone therapy improves a number of intermediate outcomes and cardiac risk factors. With the exception of the TOM trial (Testosterone in Older Men with Mobility Limitations), a study conducted in older, frail men with a high prevalence of cardiovascular disease, these trials and subsequent meta-analyses did not demonstrate adverse cardiovascular outcomes in men on testosterone replacement therapy.

- A clinical trial evaluating the effect of testosterone therapy on cardiovascular outcomes including mortality, MI, and stroke has not been conducted to my knowledge.

- The association between testosterone therapy use and adverse outcomes observed in this study differs from the association observed in a prior retrospective VA study. In the study by Shores et al, investigators noted a 39% reduction in mortality risk among patients treated with testosterone therapy.

- Elderly men with low serum testosterone levels have an increased risk of mortality and subjects with low values of both testosterone and estradiol levels have the highest risk of mortality (Journal of Clinical Endocrinology and Metabolism 94: 2482-2488, 2009)

So what does this mean exactly? We know definitively that optimized testosterone levels are associated improved health, higher quality of life and with lower rates of death. Additionally, testosterone replacement therapy improves sexual function, cognitive function, lipid profiles, endothelial function, muscle mass, free fat mass, exercise capacity, strength and endurance. Currently, the risk/benefit ratio analysis for the use of Testosterone Replacement Therapy in testosterone deficient men is highly favorable. I would encourage you if you are on testosterone replacement therapy to have a discussion with your physician or a physician knowledgeable in testosterone replacement therapy.

The media has done men in general a disservice with their usual dramatization of the story and often-misguided interpretation, which leads to confusion and misplaced trust. If you are on Testosterone Replacement Therapy, I still strongly recommend the use of Testosterone Replacement Therapy to improve your overall health profile, accompanied by appropriate monitoring laboratory, follow up, therapeutic lifestyle adjustments, exercise, and physician management. So then why do some men on testosterone have heart attacks or strokes? It's not because they are on testosterone. It's because they have undetected heart disease and heart disease is the number 1 silent killer of both men and women. One out of 3.5 men will die from heart disease. Every decade we age our risk for heart attacks and strokes rise dramatically. If you have preexisting heart disease than your risk for a secondary event is even higher.

In the weeks BEFORE a Heart Attack 95% of people suffer from these symptoms; do you suffer from any of these symptoms?

- Unusual Fatigue
- Unusual Sweating
- Shortness of Breath
- Shoulder Pain
- Neck Pain
- Difficulty Walking Upstairs or to the Mailbox
- Indigestion
- Chest Pain
- Weakness
- Sleep Disturbance
- Feeling Lightheaded or Passing Out
- Feeling like Something Bad is About to Happen

At the time of a Heart Attack people commonly have symptoms of:

- Shortness of Breath 60%
- Cheat Pain 57%
- Weakness 55%
- Fatigue 43%

Other Presenting Symptoms at Time of Heart Attack;

- Upper Abdominal Pain
- Abdominal Fullness
- Abdominal Burning Sensation
- Nausea
- Neck, Back, and/or Jaw Pain
- Feeling of Impending Doom

As we age the prevalence of heart disease increases substantially each decade!

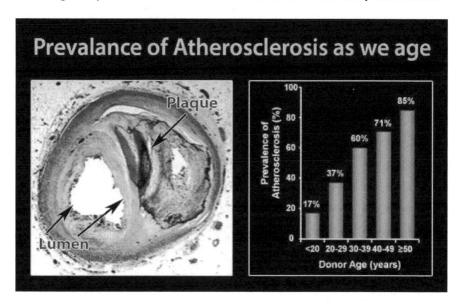

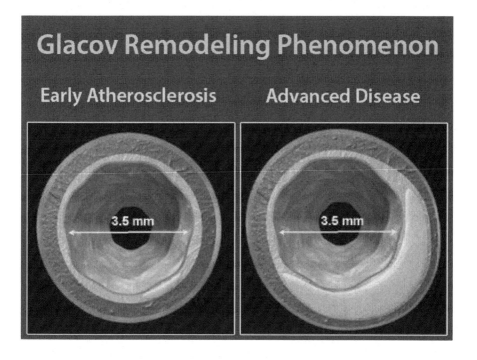

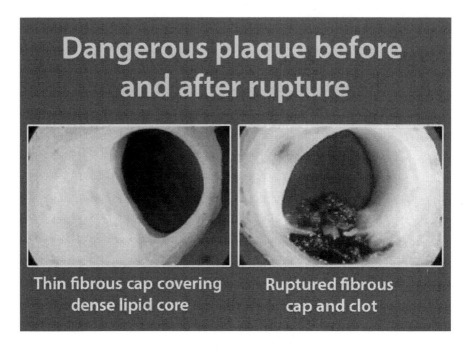

Dangerous plaque before and after rupture

Thin fibrous cap covering dense lipid core

Ruptured fibrous cap and clot

Heart disease quietly waiting to strike!

Sudden plaque rupture and heart attack! Over 50% of people having a heart attack have so called "Normal Cholesterol"!

Identifying hidden, active cardiovascular inflammatory disease can make the difference between life and death! Standard cholesterol testing and outdated Risk Assessment Scores will NOT discover your silent heart attack risk. Over 50% of all heart attacks happen in individuals with so-called "normal cholesterol". Before considering testosterone replacement therapy, you must actively seek out hidden cardiovascular disease. What difference will it make if you correct your low testosterone but don't address the possible hidden underlying cardiac threat to your life?

In one particular study researchers discovered that these 3 risk factors; low free testosterone, low high-density lipoprotein (HDL, the good cholesterol), and increasing age where strong predictors of severe coronary artery disease. While not smoking, maintaining normal blood pressures, controlling cholesterol levels, and maintaining a low glycemic state are all positive steps to preventing heart disease there is more that can be done.

In another study published by the American Heart Association, carotid ultrasounds were used to measure the thickness of the carotid arteries located in the neck. What was discovered was that men with low free testosterone levels had a 3.5 times greater progression of the thickening of the carotid artery than men with higher free testosterone levels. What this means to you is a greater chance of having a stroke.

Controlling your blood sugar levels is a step that will not only help raise your free testosterone level but also slow the process of aging and protect the cardiovascular system from disease and dangerous atherosclerosis. One study found that men with elevated hemoglobin A1c also had lower levels of free testosterone, which increased their risk for heart attacks and strokes.

What you need to have done:

1. Specialized Laboratory including:

- NMR Lipoprotein Particles NOT calculated particles!
- Inflammation Oxidation Profile
- Myocardial Stress Profile
- Lipoprotein Genetics
- Coagulation Genetics
- Renal Genetics
- Hs-Omega-3 Index
- Metabolic Profiles

2. Specialized Examinations including:

- VENDYS testing
- Carotid Ultrasound with CIMT
- Ankle-Brachial Index Testing
- VO2 Max Testing
- DEXA Scan
- Cardiac Stress Testing
- CT angiogram
- CT calcium score

Below are the laboratory tests you need to help identify your true cardio-metabolic-stroke risk.

Inflammation Oxidation

- Myeloperoxidase: is an enzyme made by white blood cells. High level is a sign of surface inflammation of the artery wall. Elevated MPO levels are associated with future risk of coronary artery disease, heart failure, heart attack, and stroke in otherwise healthy individuals.
- Lp-PLA2: elevations of this enzyme indicate serious inflammation in artery walls that can be dangerous when blood pressure is also high.
- hs-CRP: identifies inflammation in the body.
- Fibrinogen Activity: high levels of this protein mean you are at risk of developing a blood clot.

Lipoprotein Genetics

- Apo E Genotype: identifies how people respond to dietary fat and how they carry cholesterol in the blood. Apo E comes in different types, E3 is desirable, E2 is borderline, and E4 is undesirable.

Lipoprotein Particles

- NMR Lipid Profile: clinically reliable test to measure lipoproteins.
- Lipoprotein Insulin Resistance Score: insulin resistance is the precursor to diabetes and manifests its earliest measurable abnormality through changes in lipoproteins.
- LDL-P: the actual number of *bad* cholesterol particles in your blood
- HDL-P: the actual number of *good* cholesterol particles in your blood
- Lp (a): is the worst form of LDL and is an inherited trait that can increase the risk of heart attack and stroke.

Myocardial Stress

- Galectin-3: high levels of this carbohydrate binding protein contribute to abnormal thickening and stiffening of the heart muscle and change the heart structure.
- NT-proBNP: stress or strain on your heart can cause levels of this peptide to rise. If your levels are high your heart is being overworked.

Coagulation Genetics

- Factor V Leiden Mutation: this factor helps to identify if you are at risk for forming blood clots.
- Prothrombin Mutation: this factor helps to identify if you are at risk for forming blood clots.
- MTHFR: this gene provides your body with instructions to make a protein responsible for folate metabolism. This helps to assess your risk for coronary artery disease and stroke and which medication may be best for you.

Renal

- Cystatin C: is used as a biomarker of kidney function. High levels indicate a decline in kidney function.

Hs-omega-3 index

- RBC EPA+ DHA: these fatty acids are important constituents of cell membranes in our body and are vital to your cardiovascular health.

Metabolic

- Free Fatty Acid: elevated FFA level can impair your body's response to insulin and cause your blood glucose levels to rise. Higher FFA levels are a precursor to insulin resistance.
- Glucose: excess glucose in the blood can lead to diabetes and may long term complications.
- 25-hydrox-Vitamin D: long-term studies have linked vitamin D deficiency with a twofold-increased risk of heart attack and cardiovascular events.
- Homocysteine: high levels of this amino acid can injure blood vessel walls.
- Vitamin B12 & Folate: your body needs these vitamins to make blood cells and maintain a healthy nervous system.
- HbA1c: levels indicate how well your blood glucose has been controlled over the last 3-4 months. High levels indicate risk for the development of diabetes.

- Adiponectin: is a protein produced by body fat that protects against insulin resistance and inflammation. Adiponectin levels are low in those who are overweight. If you have low adiponectin levels you are at greater risk for diabetes and heart disease.
- Ferritin: is a protein that binds iron and transports it through the bloodstream. High ferritin levels can indicate problems with your body's ability to store iron. Increased ferritin levels also occur when inflammation or insulin resistance is present in your body indicating an increased risk of diabetes and heart disease.
- Alpha-hydroxybutyrate: is a small molecule produced by the liver during energy production. High levels of alpha-hydroxybutyrate are a early indicator of insulin resistance.
- Linoleoyl-glycerophosphocholine (L-GPC): low levels are an early sign of insulin resistance.
- Insulin: is a hormone responsible for regulating blood glucose levels. High levels of insulin may indicate a problem with your body's ability to control blood sugar.
- C-peptide: is a small protein that is released when insulin is created from proinsulin.
- Proinsulin: insulin is created from a non-active form called proinsulin. High levels of proinsulin may be early signs of damage to your beta cells of the pancreas.
- Anti-GAD: is a type of antibody that is created when your beta cells are being attacked by your immune system.

In a study conducted by Dr. Charles Glueck of the Jewish Hospital Cholesterol and Metabolism Center, his research found that men who developed blood clots after starting testosterone therapy, not one of the men knew previously that they had an inherited clotting disorder that put them at greater risk of developing a blood clot.

Dr. Glueck stated in an interview; "The incidence of DVT-PE or other clots in men on testosterone therapy is not known, but our best estimates are that about 1-2% of men taking testosterone will develop blood clots related to underlying inherited clotting abnormalities or to acquired thrombophilia, the antiphospholipid antibody syndrome."

"These men who landed in the hospital with dangerous and potentially lethal blood clots in the deep veins of the legs or in the lungs developed these clots within three months of starting testosterone therapy. None of them knew previously that they had an inherited clotting disorder that put them at greater risk for developing clots, nor did their providers test them before putting them on testosterone therapy."

Dr. Glueck suggests all men should have a simple blood test to determine whether they are at high risk for blood clots before starting testosterone replacement therapy.

If you have a history of a previous thromboembolism (blood clots), a family history of an inherited blood clotting disorder or are not sure then you should consider these labs as well.

- Factor V Leiden mutation
- Factor VIII
- Factor XI
- Factor II (Prothrombin gene)

Before you start testosterone replacement therapy insist on a complete cardio-metabolic workup that includes laboratory as well as screening of the cardiovascular system. Then ensure you get appropriate monitoring laboratory, make therapeutic lifestyle adjustments, get regular exercise, stop smoking, stop eating excessive sugar, and maintain follow up and physician management. Remember, you are the commander of your own health.

Low T Patient Profile: **What's Binding You Up?**

48 year old dentist, professional male with a 3-year history of growing persistent fatigue, lethargy, altered sleep, losing muscle, decreased libido, and poor erectile quality. Also senses a decreased enjoyment in life and inability to make it through the day without the need for constant caffeine.

DXA: Excellent bone mineralization, body composition 16% free fat mass
VO2: Excellent results
Neurocognitive evaluation: Decreased executive function and verbal memory
Carotid Ultrasound with CIMT: No signs of plaque or thickening
VENDYS Testing: Good to excellent

Labs:

Glucose: 89mg/dL
HgA1c: 5.1
Liver panel: normal
CBC: normal
PSA: 0.9
Insulin: 8.0uIU/mL
Lipid Panel: normal
Prolactin: 6.0
Cortisol AM: 16
LH: 5.0 mIU/mL
Total Testosterone: 533ng/dL

Free Testosterone: 5.9pg/mL
Sensitive Estradiol: 9.0pg/mL
DHT: 48ng/dL
SHBG: 74.0nmol/L!
DHEA Sulfate: 230/dL
Vitamin D: 40.2ng/mL
Serum Iron: 123ug/dL
Serum Ferritin: 195ng/mL
TSH: 1.0 uIU/mL
fT3: 3.8 pg/mL
fT4: 1.09 ng/dL

Physical Examination revealed:

Obviously fatigued appearance, but well-nourished with poor muscle structure
Normal blood pressure 118/74
Average testicles
DRE: unremarkable

Considerations for Differential Diagnosis:

Androgen Deficiency secondary to Excessive SHBG
DHEA Deficiency
Vitamin D deficiency
Zinc deficient by Zinc Tally Test
Excessive Caffeine Intake

Therapy and Recommendations:

10 Day Liver Detoxification along with a Mediterranean diet
Nettle Root 300mg three times daily
Testralin two daily
Zinc 75 mg two daily
Omega 10 one daily
Vitamin D 5000IU Sublingual QD
DHEA 25mg twice daily
8 oz. warm water with Sea Salt QAM
No Alcohol
No caffeine
Restorative Sleep in bed by 10PM

Subjective Patient Report

Feels drastic improvement inside 10-day period
No longer feels the need to have coffee

Follow Up Lab at 90 days:

Liver panel: normal
CBC: normal
Lipid Panel: normal
Prolactin: 6.0
Cortisol AM: 17.0
LH: 4.0 mIU/mL
Total Testosterone: 782ng/dL
Free Testosterone: 17.0pg/mL
Sensitive Estradiol: 14.6pg/mL

DHT: 68ng/dL
SHBG: 32.0nmol/L
DHEA Sulfate: 379.0ug/dL
Vitamin D: 60.2ng/mL
Serum Iron: 145ug/dL
Serum Ferritin: 195ng/mL
TSH: 1.0 uIU/mL
fT3: 3.7 pg/mL
fT4: 1.09 ng/dL

Take Home Point

Investigate the cause of the hypogonadism and correct underlying deficiencies and excesses before committing yourself to a therapy that is not clinically needed… Just Yet!

Chapter 5

Exhaust Natural Ways of Elevating Testosterone First

Testosterone Restoration Therapy

A 2010 study concluded that besides aging alone that lifestyle and different comorbidities were associated with total testosterone decline suggesting that age related total testosterone decline could be partially prevented by the management of risk factors and adjusting lifestyle related health behaviors.

Testosterone in the major sex hormone in the human body. Its production starts in the brain and ends in the testes in men and the ovaries in women. The adrenal glands located on top of the kidneys also produce testosterone in limited amounts. The brain and the testes work in concert to keep production in the normal range. When testosterone levels are low the brain signals the testes to make more and when there is enough testosterone, the byproducts of testosterone production signal the brain to stop. The regulation of this production referred to as the Hypothalamic-Pituitary-Testicular Axis can be disrupted at any point causing either primary or secondary hypogonadism. Provided you have and intact H-P-T axis and sufficient leydig cell function in the testes to produce testosterone in the first place these twelve testosterone restoration therapy tips can help boost cellular communication and your body's natural production of testosterone.

1. Eat Healthy Fats

The consumption of healthy fats encourages and is necessary for the production of adequate testosterone while a low fat diet will reduce testosterone levels. Healthy fat is so important that it is used by all the cells in the body to construct the cellular membrane and it serves as the source material from which testosterone is made. Research has demonstrated that a diet with less than 40% fat will lead to a decrease in testosterone levels.

Consume these healthy fats on a regular basis to ensure hormone production:

- Flaxseed (better than flax oil)
- Avocado
- Olive oil
- Green Leafy Vegetables
- Salmon, Tuna, Trout, Sardines (long chain omega-3)
- Walnuts
- Almonds
- Pistachios

If you like the supplementation route instead, be sure to choose long chain omega-3 fats from seafood sources as these provide a rich source of omega-3 and are also associated with decreased rate of sudden death.

Benefits of Fish Oil:

- Increased nitric oxide production
- Reduce triglyceride levels by 20-30%
- Improve cell membrane flexibility
- Improved insulin sensitivity
- Associated with increased cognitive function
- Decreased endothelial cytokine levels
- Decreased platelet activation
- Decrease inflammation
- Decrease clot formation
- Inhibition of ICAM and VCAM markers of endothelial dysfunction

Daily supplementation requires 1 gram per day, which is equal to 3 servings of fish per week. The best seafood sources are salmon, sardines, trout, shrimp, and crab. If you suffer from metabolic syndrome, arrhythmias, or wish to decrease your dementia risk then supplement with 1 gram per day. If you suffer from high triglycerides or inflammatory conditions like Rheumatoid Arthritis or Crohn's then supplement with 3 grams per day.

Keep your ratio of EPA/DHA to 60/40. EPA has greater anti-inflammatory effect and triglyceride lowering effect and also is converted to DHA. If you are taking anticoagulants, fish oil may increase your bleeding risk if you are taking greater than 2 grams per day.

2. Follow a Low Glycemic Nutrition Plan

The cornerstone of all health is nutrition. Consuming foods that cause high blood sugar spikes will drop your testosterone production and the resultant high insulin levels from the high blood sugar will compete with growth hormone for the same receptor site, making it difficult to have strong, healthy, lean muscle. There are numerous benefits to following a low glycemic nutrition plan such as having high energy levels, an efficient immune system, maintaining a healthy weight, a lean and muscular profile, control over food, and potential for increased longevity.

When a low glycemic meal is consumed, blood glucose elevates much slower and consistently which allows the pancreas to moderate insulin release. Since there is less insulin circulating in the blood stream, fewer cells absorb glucose and glucose levels never fall below an ideal range. Food cravings and low energy crashes diminish once you adjust to the low glycemic nutrition plan, as the body is consistently able to utilize body fat as its primary source of energy.

Consuming balanced low glycemic meals help to maintain a consistent balance of hormone levels which then allows the body to function in an ideal environment.

Insulin Competes with Growth Hormone

These two hormones use the same receptor site to communicate with cells and only one hormone can be "functionally" elevated at a time. Controlling your insulin levels with a low glycemic nutrition plan will allow growth hormone to be high and functional.

Healthy Glucose Levels

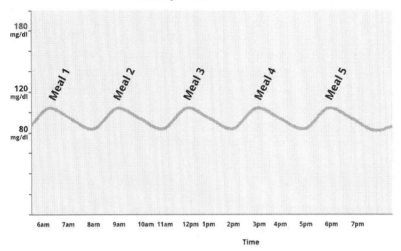

Healthy frequent meals equal steady state glucose and insulin levels, increased metabolism and decreased cravings. Steady state glucose and insulin levels equal increased fat utilization and decreased fat production.

The other side of the coin!

When processed carbohydrates are consumed, the body breaks down, absorbs, and then transports them thru the bloodstream in the form of blood glucose to the cells to be used as energy. However, most cells cannot absorb glucose without the presence of insulin. When blood glucose rises, so does insulin. This is a natural, physiological process that only becomes an issue when high glycemic foods are consumed on a regular basis.

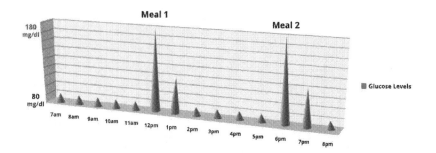

High glycemic foods increase blood glucose rapidly, resulting in high insulin levels. Insulin is a "storage" hormone. It not only promotes the absorption of sugar, but, because there is already enough free energy in the bloodstream in the form of glucose, insulin inhibits cells from releasing their stores of fatty acids. Fatty acids comprise stored fat tissue. Therefore, when insulin levels are high, the body cannot utilize body fat as an energy source.

Insulin does not immediately dissipate as glucose levels fall. In the presence of insulin, cells will continually absorb glucose, causing blood levels to fall to an unhealthy level. Because the brain can only utilize glucose for energy, food cravings and low energy become typical experiences.

Effects of a high glycemic diet:

- Erratic energy levels
- Food cravings
- Fatigue
- Weight gain
- Increased abdominal fat
- Increase in cellulite
- Decreased testosterone production

3. Supplement with Vitamin D

Vitamin D, a steroid pro-hormone, is essential for the healthy development of the nucleus of the sperm cell, and helps maintain semen quality and sperm count. Vitamin D also increases levels of testosterone, which may boost libido. In one study, overweight men who were given vitamin D supplements had a significant increase in testosterone levels after one year.

When Vitamin D levels decline during the fall and winter months, so do your testosterone levels. Supplementing with Vitamin D during these months will help ensure adequate hormone production. If you live north of Florida then you are most likely vitamin D deficient. It is the most common vitamin deficiency I see on a daily basis and the effects from supplementation are profound.

Benefits of Vitamin D:

- Increases calcium absorption
- Improves bone health
- Decreases autoimmune disease rates
- Improved Blood Pressure Control
- Lower Cardiovascular disease rate
- Blocks progression of pre-cancerous cells

Great Vitamin D Sources:

- Cod Liver Oil
- Calcium Rich Foods
- Egg Yolk
- Sunshine exposure
- Supplementation

Which should you take; Vitamin D2 or D3? Well both are converted into 25-hydroxyvitamin D, but Vitamin D3 is about 5 times more potent than Vitamin D2. The goal of Vitamin D therapy is to reach a level of at least 40-70ng/ml and the average individual needs an intake of 2,000 IU daily to reach a blood level greater than 40 ng/ml.

4. Correct your Magnesium Deficiency

An incredibly common deficiency seen in America and a 2001-2002 NHANES study demonstrated that 57% of the population is deficient. Great sources of magnesium are almonds, green leafy vegetables and avocados! Supplementation with Magnesium glycinate 200-400mg daily will do the job. Magnesium glycinate is a chelated form of magnesium that tends to provide the highest levels of absorption and bioavailability and is typically considered ideal for those who are trying to correct a deficiency.

An important note is that calcium supplementation blocks the absorption of magnesium! Current recommendations are to supplement with a 2:1 calcium/magnesium ratio, however the appropriate ratio of calcium to magnesium is 1:1. An incorrect ratio of calcium to magnesium may not only pose a risk to your bones but also to your heart. If you have too much calcium and not enough magnesium your muscles can go into spasm. Also, excessive amounts of calcium without the counterbalance of magnesium can lead to abnormal heart rhythms, coronary vasospasm and sudden death. If you are magnesium deficient, your heart simply cannot function properly, which will affect all areas of your performance.

5. Correct your Zinc Deficiency

Next to vitamin D deficiency, zinc deficiency is incredibly common. Low levels of zinc are associated with low levels of testosterone. The mineral zinc is important for testosterone production, and supplementing your diet for as little as six weeks has been shown to cause a marked improvement in testosterone among men with low levels. Zinc also inhibits aromatase, which converts testosterone into estrogen. Zinc also plays a crucial role in pituitary function and in the cellular communication process in the H-P-T axis.

Be sure to consume these foods to help boost your T levels!

- Nuts, especially cashews
- Dark chocolate
- Spinach
- Seafood like crab, lobsters, and shrimp
- Lamb
- Raw Milk, Raw Cheese

Deficiency can also be easily corrected with a high quality daily phytomultivitamin that also contains chromium and selenium. If you decide to use a zinc supplement, stick to a dosage of around 40 mg a day, as this is the recommended adult upper limit. Taking too much zinc can interfere with your body's ability to absorb other minerals.

6. Run Sprints or High Intensity Interval Training (H.I.I.T.)

Running sprints or short bursts of intensity lasting approximately 6 seconds dramatically increase the levels of testosterone and the catecholamines: adrenaline and noradrenaline.

You might be surprised to know that exercise boosts testosterone, no matter what your age. In a new study, researchers looked at both younger and older men who did 21 weeks of intense training. They measured significant increases in lean body mass and testosterone.

A HIIT session consists of a warm up period of exercise, followed by six to ten repetitions of high intensity exercise, separated by medium intensity exercise, and ending with a period of cool down exercise. The high intensity exercise should be done at near maximum intensity, 90%. The medium exercise should be about 50% intensity. The number of repetitions and length of each depends on the exercise. The goal is to do at least six cycles, and to have the entire HIIT session last between fifteen and twenty minutes. HIIT is considered to be an excellent way to maximize a fat loss workout. HIIT increases the RMR (resting metabolic rate) for the following 24 hours. HIIT turns on your metabolic fire! Specific hormones that are released during this type of training are growth hormone and catecholamines, which contribute significantly to a decrease in body fat. Catecholamines are fat destroying hormones that have been shown to liberate both intramuscular and subcutaneous fat. Steady state exercise only results in small increases in catecholamines. HIIT is a powerful stimulator of growth hormone –a hormone that limits lipoprotein lipase, which is a fat storage enzyme. Another powerful stimulator of growth hormone is getting a full night of sleep. HIIT has been extensively studied and is significantly more effective at fat reduction than steady state exercise and also increases the levels of circulating testosterone.

Exercise Pausing and Increased Fat Loss

The type and intensity of exercise you perform directly affects how adrenaline and noradrenaline are released from the adrenal glands and the nerve terminals playing a major role in fat loss - and less fat means more testosterone. This is why I'm such a fan of High Intensity Interval Training. It's short, it's fast, and it's done with great results.

Taking a closer look we see as exercise intensity goes up so does the release of adrenaline and noradrenaline. Once you cross the lactate threshold then adrenaline and noradrenaline release explode. Now after you finish a HIIT Session take a *5-minute break after your initial 20 minutes of HIIT* and rest. This is recommended because there is a large release of fatty acids into the bloodstream about 5 minutes after your HIIT training ends.

Now if we do nothing those fatty acids that were released during the 5-minute break will be *re-stored* in the fat cell and in some men, especially estrogen dominant men and women fat likes to re-store below the waist. So...that's why after your 5-minute break you get back on the treadmill and run at a slower pace about 50% effort for 10-20 minutes to utilize the free fatty acids floating in the bloodstream. Now they are gone for good and you are feeling lighter and leaner than ever and making more testosterone! This simple strategy can literally bust you through any plateau in your training yet it is one of the least utilized.

7. Lift Heavy Weight

There are numerous resistance-training programs you can follow; hypertrophy plans, strength plans, strength and endurance plans, body weight workouts, rage workouts, Fibonacci sets and more. All of these plans will cause a specific adaptation to the imposed demand. Resistance training or weight training is a potent stimulator for testosterone production. Be sure to include some form of weight training 2-3 times per week to help boost your body's natural production of testosterone. Interestingly, rest periods of 90 seconds between sets has the greatest effect on post workout testosterone and growth hormone levels.

8. Avoid Chronic Stress

It is vitally important to rest your body as well. Adequate rest promotes recuperation and recovery. Excessive training, stress, and/or inadequate amounts of sleep contribute to elevate cortisol levels, which is antagonistic to and reduces testosterone levels. Your body unfortunately will produce cortisol instead of testosterone so high exposure to stress and high levels of cortisol lead to low testosterone. This is the last thing you want when it comes to maintaining peak performance and testosterone levels. Appropriate rest and recovery also promotes healthy growth hormone levels. Also, avoid too much of a good thing. Excessive or chronic training can lead to overtraining syndrome, which is counterproductive to a balanced hormonal environment.

9. Consider Controlled Fasting for Calorie Restriction

I know, "what do you mean don't eat"? Not quite, you get to eat, it's just that we like you to eat during a specific window of time during the day and then abstain from food during a period of time when you are most likely relaxing and preparing to rest for the evening. Why is this?

Controlled fasting boosts testosterone by increasing the expression of satiety hormones including insulin, leptin, adiponectin, glucagon-like peptide-1 (GLP-1), colecystokinin (CKK) and melanocortins, all of which are known to potentiate healthy testosterone actions, increase libido and prevent age-related testosterone decline.

The substantial impact of calorie restriction on mitochondria, the little powerhouses of our cells, is rather profound as well. Clive McCay from Cornell University in the 1950's recorded an increased life expectancy of close to 35% in rats fed a calorie-restricted diet. The longest controlled study of calorie restriction on a primate has been a 25-year study at the University of Wisconsin studying the effects of calorie restriction on monkeys and the results are amazing. The calorie-restricted monkeys have demonstrated healthier profiles and life expectancy.

But what about eating breakfast? "Isn't it the most important meal of the day?" Well, breakfast just means to "break the fast" and we still are "breaking the fast" just a little later in the morning. It is still an important meal and we will get to that in just a minute.

Fasting is defined as: *An act of willingly abstaining or reduction from certain or all food, drink, or both for a period of time. An absolute fast is normally defined as abstinence from all food or liquid for a defined period, usually a single day, or several days.*

I personally use a controlled fast daily as a way of giving our bodies a break from all the digestive work and as a way of giving myself freedom from food. It's amazing how much you can accomplish when you do not have to take breaks to eat.

You may think that you'll have no energy and that you will starve. But, quite the opposite happens. Your energy levels and productivity will skyrocket! You will more than likely feel unbelievably energized too! You have more than enough energy stored in your body to exist for this very brief period, 12-18 hours without solid food. During this controlled fast I drink plenty of water with lemon to stay well hydrated. Also at any time during this period, you are in control, you can choose to end your controlled fast whenever you like and still amazing benefits.

It's easiest to start with the simplest controlled fast, the 6pm to 6 am. You are asleep for most of this 12-hour period; you should be hitting the rack around 10 p.m. Then work your way to a 16-18 hour fast. You are always in control and can choose to end your fast whenever you like. When you choose to eat, remember to eat appropriately and not overeat. Chances are you will feel full quickly even with a small amount of food.

Planned Controlled Fasting Schedules:

Schedule 1: 6pm to 6am (the easiest)
Schedule 2: 6pm to 10 am (move from a 12 hour to 16-18 hour)
Schedule 3: 6pm to Noon
Schedule 4: 8pm to Noon
Schedule 5: Any 16-18 hour period that fits your schedule.

Short-term fasting has been shown to have the following health benefits, which were found after as little as 12-24 hours of fasting!

- Decreased body fat & body weight
- Maintenance of skeletal muscle mass
- Decreased blood glucose levels
- Increased glucagon levels
- Increased lipolysis & fat oxidation
- Decreased insulin levels & increased insulin sensitivity
- Increased cellular cleansing
- Increased norepinephrine & epinephrine levels
- Increased growth hormone levels
- Decreased food related stress
- Decreased chronic systemic Inflammation

These are all drinks that would be allowed during your fast:

- Black Coffee
- Green tea
- Herbal tea
- Water
- Sparkling Water

So what happens when you fast?

During the first 24 hours of fasting circulating glucose, fatty acids, triglycerides, and liver and muscle glycogen are used as energy sources. However, the total of these energy stores in the average 70kg man is about 1200 kcal. And this is less energy than is needed for basal metabolism for a 24 hour period. Glucose from the liver is derived from hepatic glycogen and since there is only about 70 grams of glycogen in the average human liver, glycogenolysis can only sustain glucose levels for about 8-10 hours in the presence of exercise this period is even shorter. To compensate for the depletion of glycogen, gluconeogenesis begins with a flux of substrate from muscle and fat stores to the liver and to sites for utilization. Glycerol released from fat stores and lactate, pyruvate and alanine derived from muscle are the precursors for hepatic glucose synthesis.

Triglycerides that come from adipose tissue can be catabolized into fatty acids and ketone bodies by most tissues. However over the short run tissues such as the brain can only use glycolytic pathways to obtain energy. Since the conversion of fatty acids to carbohydrate is insufficient, these glycolytic tissues must utilize either glucose or substrates that can be converted to glucose. Amino acids derived primarily from skeletal muscle constitute the major endogenous substrate for glucose production for this purpose. Since there is no storage form of protein in the body, a long-term (>24 hours) fasting individual will sustain a daily loss of functional protein.

The provision of adequate fuel substrate to critical tissue, particularly the brain, has priority during energy deprivation or fasting. Brief periods of fasting lead to acute adaptive responses that sustain the supply of glucose to the tissues that require it and to minimize the amount of protein breakdown to meet this need. To accomplish this, certain tissues such as the heart, kidneys, and skeletal muscle change their primary fuel source from glucose to fatty acids and ketone bodies. Other tissues such as bone marrow, renal medulla and peripheral nerves switch from full oxidation of glucose to anaerobic glycolysis, which results in the production of lactate and pyruvate.

These compounds can be converted to glucose in the liver with energy derived from fat oxidation and then released for consumption. The Cori cycle enables energy stored as fat to be utilized for glucose synthesis and thus conserves protein energy that would otherwise be necessary for the new synthesis of glucose.

Anabolic phase (a few hours after the meal)

- Primary hormone is insulin
- Plasma substrates are increased glucose, triglycerides, branch chained amino acids, and a decrease in free fatty acids and ketones.
- Active process is glycogen storage, protein synthesis, and triglyceride production.

Catabolic phase (about 5-6 hours after a meal)

- Initiated by fall in insulin.
- Primary hormone is glucagon.
- Plasma substrates are a decrease in glucose, triglycerides and an increase in alanine and glutamine, free fatty acids, and ketones.

Active processes are glycogenolysis, gluconeogenesis, proteolysis, lipolysis, ketogenesis. Once the body has digested, stored, and metabolized your last meal, it begins utilizing the many options in meeting your energy requirements and optimizing hormone levels. Your body is then busy using all of the stored energy sources, which means you are losing weight, decreasing inflammation, stabilizing hormones, and increasing cellular cleansing. Short periods of fasting 12-18 hours will provide incredible health benefits for you over the short and long term and give you control over food.

10. Eat Red Meat

Eating lean red meat will not kill you. However, low testosterone from not eating red meat just might. A study of vegans vs. omnivores measured each group's testosterone and SHBG. The vegans had 23% higher SHBG and 3% lower free testosterone, not a good combination for manliness. Red meat contains saturated fat, which has a strong correlation with higher testosterone and zinc that helps you produce testosterone. Choose free-range grass feed beef because it has more B vitamins. B vitamins help your body to make testosterone and absorb zinc so you can make more testosterone.

I tried a vegan diet for approximately 2 weeks, it actually was quite invigorating and I did notice several benefits such as clearer skin and better reading vision. However, I did notice a decrease in my endurance and strength by the end of the second week. Going into the vegan diet my total testosterone was 810 ng/dL and Free T was 16.9 pg/dL with a SHBG of 44 nmol/L. After the 2-week period my levels had plummeted to a TT of 511 ng/dL, FT of 7.0 pg/dL, and SHBG of 60 nmol/L. Needless to say but a 1-½ inch porterhouse steak with organic butter hit a hot cast iron skillet that night! No more veganism for this guy.

11. Lower Your Estrogen Level

As men grow older they produce more aromatase. As a result more testosterone is converted into estrogen. While normal levels of estrogen are necessary and beneficial to men for their overall health, excess estrogen can lead to feminizing effects, narrowing of coronary arteries, increasing clotting factors, and crashing a man's libido. Being overweight, drinking too much alcohol, aging, zinc deficiency, consuming estrogen-producing foods, genetic predisposition, and exposure to endocrine disruptors can all play a role in increasing estrogen levels. Consequently as estrogen levels raise so does the level of SHBG (Sex Hormone Binding Globulin), which preferentially binds more testosterone and further increases estrogen levels. It is a vicious cycle. Unfortunately the direct manipulation of the SHBG level is not an easy or predictable task. Many a man with a functional H-P-T axis has been effectively neutered by having their free testosterone nearly completely bound by an age related increase in SHBG.

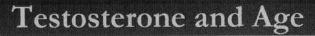

Testosterone and Age

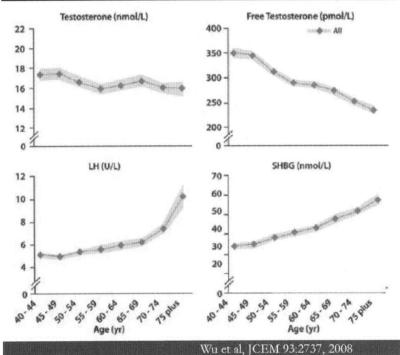

Wu et al, JCEM 93:2737, 2008

So what can you do to lower your estrogen level?

- Correct any zinc deficiency
- Maintain a lean body mass
- Limit or eliminate alcohol consumption
- Remove endocrine disrupting chemicals
- Consume a cruciferous vegetable with every meal
- Promote liver health and its detoxification pathways
- Use estrogen lowering supplements if necessary

12. Check Your Intracellular Nutrient Status

Overwhelming scientific evidence has substantiated that vitamin deficiencies are associated with multiple disease processes and the overall condition of an individuals' health. Vitamin, mineral and antioxidant deficiencies have been shown to not only suppress immune function but also contribute to chronic degenerative diseases such as arthritis, cancer, dementia, cardiovascular disease, diabetes, and hormone deficiencies

In particular low levels of vitamin D and low free testosterone levels are both associated with increased mortality. Studies show an intricate association between vitamin D and androgen metabolism suggesting that a deficiency of both hormones may be associated with adverse clinical outcomes.

This brings us to the necessity of precision testing with personalized precision health care. While making all of the above adjustments to your lifestyle and nutrition is commendable and will certainly help you optimize your personal hormone status, knowing instead of guessing will always deliver better results. This is why I strongly recommend having and intracellular nutrient test performed. They are relatively inexpensive and the health information you gain is invaluable. This test is available at Spectracell Laboratories and through the Alpha Male Medical Institute.

On the following page is the intracellular nutrient test of a patient with three significant deficiencies that are related to infertility, immune function, protein synthesis, energy metabolism, fatigue, cellular communication, cellular integrity, detoxification, hormone regulation, hypogonadism, and more.

Knowing this critical information allows your physician to make precise adjustments to your supplementation. This is much better than a "shotgun" approach to vitamin and mineral supplementation, which is what most individuals do with little or no success.

Micronutrients	Patient Results (% Control)	Functional Abnormals	Reference Range (greater than)
B Complex Vitamins			
Vitamin B1 (Thiamin)	101		>78%
Vitamin B2 (Riboflavin)	58		>53%
Vitamin B3 (Niacinamide)	99		>80%
Vitamin B6 (Pyridoxine)	71		>54%
Vitamin B12 (Cobalamin)	21		>14%
Folate	40		>32%
Pantothenate	12		>7%
Biotin	51		>34%
Amino Acids			
Serine	34		>30%
Glutamine	58		>37%
Asparagine	43		>39%
Metabolites			
Choline	27		>20%
Inositol	71		>58%
Carnitine	62		>46%
Fatty Acids			
Oleic Acid	67		>65%
Other Vitamins			
Vitamin D3 (Cholecalciferol)	55		>50%
Vitamin A (Retinol)	78		>70%
Vitamin K2	70		>30%
Minerals			
Calcium	34	Deficient	>38%
Manganese	59		>50%
Zinc	36	Deficient	>37%
Copper	55		>42%
Magnesium	52		>37%
Carbohydrate Metabolism			
Glucose-Insulin Interaction	51		>38%
Fructose Sensitivity	37		>34%
Chromium	44		>40%
Antioxidants			
Glutathione	38	Deficient	>42%
Cysteine	53		>41%
Coenzyme Q-10	95		>86%
Selenium	82		>74%
Vitamin E (A-tocopherol)	91		>84%
Alpha Lipoic Acid	89		>81%
Vitamin C	59		>40%
SPECTROX™			
Total Antioxidant Function	50		>40%
Proliferation Index			
Immunidex	59		>40%

Analysis of this individual reveals these particular deficiencies and their impact to his overall health and vitality.

Calcium

Calcium is the most abundant mineral in the body, with 99% residing in bones and teeth. As a component of hard tissues, calcium fulfills a structural role to maintain body size and act as attachments for musculoskeletal tissues. The remaining 1% of calcium is present in blood and soft tissues. Functions of non-skeletal calcium include: enzyme activation, second messenger roles (transmitting hormonal information), blood clotting, cell and cell organelle membrane function (stabilization and transport), nerve impulse transmission, and muscular contraction, tone, and irritability. Calcium levels in the blood are maintained within very strict limits by dietary intake, hormonal regulation, and a rapidly exchangeable pool in bone tissue.

Zinc

The primary role of zinc is to activate almost 200 enzymes with vital roles in cell regulation, immune function, acid/base balance, DNA, RNA, and protein synthesis, lipid metabolism, eicosanoid production, and digestion. Zinc also is a component of insulin (energy metabolism), thymic hormones (immune function) and gustin (taste acuity).

Glutathione

Glutathione is implicated in many cellular functions including antioxidant protection and detoxification. It is also essential for the maintenance of cell membrane integrity in red blood cells. Intracellular glutathione concentrations are principally derived by intracellular synthesis, as few cells directly uptake glutathione from the surrounding extracellular fluid. The high concentration of glutathione in virtually all cells clearly indicates its importance in metabolic and oxidative detoxification processes. Glutathione may be considered the "preeminent" antioxidant.

For many of us, despite following all of these recommendations, you may still suffer from testosterone deficiency from one of the many causes or conditions:

- Viral Infection
- Radiation/Chemotherapy
- Genetic conditions
- Leydig cell dysfunction
- Various Medications
- Excessive Alcohol
- Aging
- Hemochromatosis
- Chronic Systemic Disease
- Diabetes
- Chronic Obstructive Pulmonary Disease
- Metabolic Syndrome
- Tumors
- Environmental Toxins

Testosterone deficiency is associated with the onset and/or worsening of these medical conditions:

- Cardiovascular disease
- Dementia
- Bone demineralization
- Joint & Tendon degeneration
- Diabetes & Metabolic Syndrome
- Depression
- Vascular endothelial dysfunction
- Increased CIMT and vaso-reactivity
- Obesity

If you are following a healthy nutrition plan, exercising regularly, drinking plenty of water, getting adequate rest and recovery but are still noticing these symptoms, then you may be suffering from testosterone deficiency despite doing all the right things:

- Poor memory, concentration, or focus
- Moody or depressed
- Lack of motivation or drive
- Lack of stamina
- Poor recovery or increased recovery time from exercise
- Loss of muscle mass or difficulty maintaining muscle mass
- Increasing belly fat or difficulty losing belly fat despite exercising
- Fatigue especially in the afternoon or after eating
- Poor libido
- Decreasing erectile quality
- Loss of hair or reduced shaving
- Hot flushes or sweats

The first step is to get the correct lab work and have a physician experienced and knowledgeable in the diagnosis, treatment, and management of male hormone deficiencies and all of its various nuisances and intricacies.

Testosterone deficiency presents with a recognizable symptom complex that is highly amenable to hormone therapy if a reliable and predictable treatment plan is consistently administered.

Testosterone is supremely important for the health and vitality of men and women. Optimizing its production by following these ten vital steps will help to ensure your personal health and well-being.

As you may come to notice in all of my writings there is always mention of the pillars of human existence that support the foundational principles of all human health. Those pillars Nutrition, Exercise, Water, Rest, Recovery and Hormone Optimization and must be cared for daily to ensure your personal health and fitness. We may not be able to stop Mother Nature but we sure can try and slow her down!

PUTTING IT TOGETHER

1. Perform your screening labs to obtain your baseline biomarkers and to check the status of your hypothalamic-pituitary-testicular axis.
2. Perform Intracellular Nutrient Testing and correct your personal deficiencies.
3. Perform Food Sensitivity Testing and eliminate your personal food sensitivities from your diet to decrease immune system response and inflammation.
4. Follow the low glycemic-nutrient timed-controlled fasting nutrition plan.
5. No Alcohol
6. Practice sleep hygiene
7. Limit caffeine intake
8. If you are contemplating having a vasectomy-DO NOT DO IT!
9. Strategically exercise
10. Follow the aforementioned recommendations in Chapter Five

DR. ROB'S Fast Five Supplements for Boosting Testosterone Naturally

This is a base supplementation plan that is a great place to start until all of your testing is completed and you can begin to personalize your supplementation strategies.

Testralin™: two tablets twice daily
Tribulus Synergy®: two tablets twice daily
Omegagenics™ Mega 10™: one tablet twice daily
Zinc A.G.™: one tablet daily
Endura®: one scoop daily during exercise

These supplements can help to naturally increase your testosterone and take you to the next level but none of these supplements are as important as following the basic foundations of human health and wellness. *Eating healthy nutrition, regular meaningful exercise, drinking plenty of water, and getting appropriate periods of rest and sleep are the foundations of human health.*

I encourage you to talk with your Doctor about any and all of the supplements you wish to start taking.

All of the supplements listed in this chapter are available in our store
http://www.alphamaleinstitute.com/the-alpha-male-store/

* These statements have not been evaluated by the Food and Drug Administration. These products are not intended to diagnose, treat, cure, or prevent any disease.

Chapter 6

Boost Testosterone by Avoiding These Items

1. Avoid Soy and Soy based products

- Soy contains phytoestrogens called isoflavones that mimic the activity of the hormone estrogen in your body.
- Soy contains goitrogens, substances that depresses thyroid function, which lead to reduced anabolic hormone production in men of all ages.
- The extremely high phytate content of soy inhibits the absorption of calcium, magnesium, iron and zinc from foods. These nutrients are absolutely critical for optimal male hormone production and testicle function.

2. Avoid ingesting Fluoride

- Fluoride is more toxic than lead, but slightly less toxic than arsenic.
- May cause severe dental fluorosis and crippling fluorosis
- Can cause arthritic symptoms and bone fracture well before the onset of crippling fluorosis, and can affect many other tissues besides bone and teeth, including the brain and thyroid gland. There is also evidence that links fluoride to a serious form of bone cancer known as osteosarcoma.
- Prolonged exposure to varying levels of fluoride can damage the brain, particularly when coupled with an iodine deficiency or aluminum excess and 37 human studies link moderately high fluoride exposures with reduced intelligence (IQ).
- Evidence of several types indicates that fluoride affects normal endocrine function
- Studies have found that high-fluoride exposure is associated with reduced male testosterone levels.
- Research shows that consumption of fluoride is linked to numerous health conditions including a common condition called hypothyroidism.

3. Avoid BPA's (Bisphenol A & B)

- Fat Producing Chemical Infused into Plastics that mimics Estrogen
- Originally developed as a estrogen replacement
- Bisphenol-A is a xenoestrogen associated with various reproductive disorders in animals
- BPA has also now been linked to heart disease, obesity, diabetes and liver dysfunction. One recent study shows that those with Bisphenol-A tissue levels in the top 25% were twice as likely to suffer from heart disease.
- Dangerous residue levels of Bisphenol-A have also now been found in an abundance of paper products. This includes just about every paper product imaginable including "napkins, toilet paper, tickets, food wrappers, newspapers, and printer paper." These levels are much higher than even those found in canned goods and can be absorbed through the skin. Receipts are particularly risky.
- Never heat food in plastic containers, especially in the microwave
- Do not put hot liquids into plastics

4. Avoid Soaps and Shampoos that contain:

- Ingredients ending in Paraben
- Sodium Lauryl Sulfate - Once it has been absorbed, one of the main effects of sodium lauryl sulfate is to mimic the activity of the hormone Oestrogen and may be responsible for a variety of health problems including a reduction in male fertility.
- Sodium Laureth Sulfate (SLES) - somewhat less irritating than SLS, but it cannot be metabolized by the liver and its effects are therefore much longer lasting.
- Propylene Glycol - slightly toxic to the skin and eyes and is toxic in large doses if ingested. The compound is absorbed through the skin, meaning that large surface exposures result in symptoms similar to those produced through ingestion. In particular, propylene glycol causes damage to the central nervous system, which includes the brain and spinal cord.

5. Avoid products that contain Phthalates

- Chemicals found in large quantity mostly in flexible plastics but also used in hundreds of agricultural, commercial, residential and consumer products.
- Common Abbreviations: DBP, DEP, DEHP, BzBP, DMP
- 1982 study showed that phthalates shunted testosterone-boosting zinc away from the testes and a study a few years later verified this and noted actual testicular atrophy (shrinkage).
- Other symptoms linked to phthalates include:
- Feminization in males
- Lowered Testosterone.
- Lowered Fertility - linked to lowered sperm quality and DNA damage
- ADHD
- Altered thyroid function
- Insulin Resistance and Diabetes.

6. Avoid foods containing High-Fructose Corn Syrup

- HFCS is broken-down by the liver, which can lead to health problems such as fatty liver, and it has also been proven that the liver converts fructose into fat far easier than it does natural sucrose.
- The human body can digest natural sugar more easily than high fructose corn syrup
- HFCS takes longer for the body to digest and rises insulin levels higher than natural sugars which can lead to a higher risk of developing diabetes

7. Avoid foods containing Butylated Hydroxyanisole (BHA)

- Used in foods such as chips, sausages and cereals as a preservative and stabilize.
- Classified as a human carcinogen and may cause an increased risk of cancer
- BHA is an endocrine interrupter and negatively affects the endocrine system and has detrimental effects on development and reproductive, immune and neurological functions.

8. Avoid foods containing Nitrates

- Used to preserve color and flavor in cured meats and fish
- Research has found that Nitrates may be the cause an increased risk of heart disease by 42% and type-2 diabetes by 19%.

9. Avoid the ingestion of Atrazine

- Atrazine is the most commonly detected pesticide contaminant of ground water, surface water, and precipitation.
- Atrazine is an endocrine disruptor that, among other effects, alters male reproductive tissues when animals are exposed during development.
- Atrazine de-masculinizes male gonads producing testicular lesions associated with reduced germ cell numbers in teleost fish, amphibians, reptiles, and mammals, and induces partial and/or complete feminization in fish, amphibians, and reptiles.

SUPPLEMENTS THAT "MAY" BOOST TESTOSTERONE

Below is a list of Supplements that may improve hormone balance, boost testosterone, block the production of excess estrogen, improve libido, prostate health, energy, muscle recovery and decrease fat. This assumes that you have an intact and functional H-P-T Axis. Best advice is to get labs first as a baseline before starting any of these supplements and work closely in concert with your physician.

1. Silybum Marianum (Milk Thistle)

- Essential in supporting healthy liver function, and depending on the health of the liver, can help rebuild parts of it as well. In order for the prostate to remain healthy, your liver should remain in optimal condition in order to continue to effectively remove toxins from the body. Milk thistle not only protects the liver, it acts as a detoxifying agent in the body.

2. Diindolylmethane (DIM)

- A natural substance formed when the human digestive system breaks down cruciferous vegetables (broccoli, cabbage, cauliflower, etc.)
- In small amounts, it can both inhibit the aromatase enzyme (and prevent conversion of testosterone into estrogen) and it can act on more potent forms of estrogen and convert them into less potent forms; this conversion reduces the overall effects of estrogen in the body. However, taking too much DIM at once can actually induce the aromatase enzyme and act in the opposite manner and increase estrogen synthesis.
- In regards to androgen metabolism, DIM appears to be a strong antagonist in human prostate cancer cells.

3. Resveratrol

- There appears to be an increase in insulin sensitivity seen with resveratrol at doses low enough to be achieved via wine consumption, all tests currently in obese and unhealthy persons.
- A significant decrease in circulating TNFα levels have been detected with resveratrol supplementation; linked to anti-inflammatory effects of resveratrol.

4. Coleus Forskohlii

- Increase CAMP in fat cells, which increase the rate of fat loss and can make other fat burners better at fat burning.
- Shown to increase Testosterone levels in men, have some anti-cancer effects, some anti-inflammatory effects, and interacts with muscle tissue
- Increasing CAMP can in part mimic caloric restriction and exercise, as CAMP is a signal of energy deprivation or energy usage.
- Increase of testosterone observed in men not overly potent and is highly variable.

5. Phosphatidylserine (Sunflower based)

- Phosphatidylserine reduces the amount of free cortisol in your body and helps keep cortisol levels in a balanced, cyclical rhythm. Phosphatidylserine has been shown to reduce post-workout muscle soreness, hasten recovery, increase fat loss and promote muscle growth.
- No significant influence on testosterone noted with PS supplementation.

6. Mucuna Pruriens (Cowhage)

- A bean-like plant grown wild in tropical climates
- Provides a neurotransmitter pre-cursor called L-Dopa, the amino acid compound the body uses to make Dopamine.
- Healthy levels of Dopamine improve energy, mood, mental focus, and motivation.
- An increase in testosterone is seen in infertile men. It is unsure if this increase in testosterone occurs in fertile and otherwise healthy men.

7. Niacin (Vitamin B3) (Nicotinic Acid)

- Helps the body metabolize glucose from food to produce energy
- Niacin is most often touted for lowering LDL cholesterol (the bad kind), protecting against cardiovascular disease and boosting HDL cholesterol (the good kind).
- Additionally, niacin plays a role in the production of hormones, including sex-related and adrenal hormones.
- Evidence that it helps reduce atherosclerosis, or hardening of the arteries.

8. Tribulus Terrestris

- Flowering plant that is native to the temperate and tropical regions of southern Europe, Asia, Africa, and Australia.
- Supplementation stimulates androgen receptors in the brain
- In otherwise healthy males, testosterone is not influenced with supplementation of *tribulus terrestris*. There may be an increase in infertile men, but this is weak.
- In infertile men, supplementation of 6g tribulus root appears to increase rigidity of erections and improve performance (reduce anxiety while delaying ejaculation and improving orgasm.

9. Fenugreek seeds

- Indigenous to India and North Africa, Trigonella foenum-graecum, more commonly known as fenugreek, is used in traditional medicine for treating arthritis and sexual dysfunction.
- Although there is limited evidence to support an increase in testosterone, more evidence than not denies such an increase.
- Increases in libido have been noted before, which is notable due to the lack of significant influence on testosterone and possible suppression of DHT (theoretically should reduce libido, yet a large increase is seen with fenugreek)

10. Avena Sativa (Oat Straw or Panax seudoginseng)

- Used in sexual supplements is also used to treat mood and anxiety
- Used to relieve pain; and to reduce swelling, cholesterol, and blood pressure. It is also used for chest pain (angina), strokes, dizziness, and sore throat.
- May increase testosterone in infertile men, has also failed in fertile men to influence testosterone; likely a mere antioxidative effect in damaged testicles.
- An improvement in erectile dysfunction is seen with 3g of Korean Red Ginseng (fermented panax ginseng, regular panax ginseng not as well tested), which is thought to be secondary to anti-fatigue effects and improved blood flow.

11. Suma (Brazilian Ginseng)

- The dried root of Pfaffia paniculata, a plant native to the Amazonian rain forests.
- May boost the immune system and combats low energy or fatigue
- No alterations noted in serum testosterone associated with ecdysterone consumption.

12. Ashwaganda (Winter Cherry)

- A shrub cultivated in India and North America whose roots contains flavonoids and many active ingredients of the withanolide class
- Testosterone may be increased in infertile men (who have a reduction in testosterone), but there is currently no evidence to suggest an inherent testosterone boosting effect in otherwise normal men.

13. Tongkat ali (Malaysian ginseng)

- Used to treat male infertility and chronically low testosterone levels in men.
- There is no evidence to suggest an inherent testosterone boosting effect in otherwise normal men.
- Contains quassinoids such as eurycomalacton, eurycomanon, eurycomanol and has been reported to have aphrodisiac properties and to increase testosterone levels in men.
- Test results suggest that water-soluble extract of Tongkat Ali increased fat free mass, reduced body fat, and increased muscle strength and size.

14. Catuaba

- A medium-sized tree found in the Amazon forest in the northern part of Brazil
- Catuaba bark is considered a central nervous system stimulant with aphrodisiac properties and a bark decoction is used for nervousness, poor memory, and sexual weakness

15. Maca (Andean Ginseng)

- Plant grows in Peru
- Prized as a nutritious food rich in fiber, amino acids and essential fatty acids.
- Study found men who took maca for four months had a significant increase in motility, sperm count and semen volume
- No significant influences on testosterone in any tested demographic.
- Studies have shown that maca might help reduce enlargement of the prostate, a condition known as benign prostatic hyperplasia by acting on androgen receptors in the prostate, preventing the binding of hormones that fuel prostate growth.
- An increase in erection frequency has been noted in men, likely related to the libido enhancing properties.

16. Muira Puama

- Study showed that short-term effects of supplementing with Muira Puama rapidly increased blood flow to the genitals, increasing sexual function and sensations for both men and women. Long-term use of this herb showed to enhance the production of sex hormones in both male and females alike.

17. Nascent Iodine

- Nascent Iodine holds an electromagnetic charge and is iodine in its atomic form.
- May work to naturally balance the thyroid to a state of homeostasis
- Stimulates thyroid production of T3 (triiodothyronine) and T4 (thyroxine) hormones
- May help stop bromine, chlorine, and fluoride storage in the body, and slow the production of goitrogens.
- Best form of iodine to protect the body from harmful radiation exposure

18. Krill Oil

Benefits of Krill Oil:
- The Omega-3 fatty acids in krill oil are known for their anticarcinogenic properties; they also prevent cardiovascular diseases and optimize the immune system. Research has also shown that a regular intake of Omega-3 fatty acids improves memory and other brain functions.
- Krill oil is a major source of choline, which is extremely important for cellular health and early brain development. Choline is present in krill oil in the form of Phosphatidylcholine, which is very important in the formation of all cell membranes; it is also responsible for the proper communication between the brain and the various parts of our body.
- The Astaxanthin contained in krill oil is one of the most powerful antioxidants in nature. Antioxidants are known to neutralize free radicals, which can cause cancer and various other chronic diseases. Unlike most antioxidants, Astaxanthin is able to cross the blood brain-barrier, thereby protecting the brain from free radical damage.
- Regular krill oil supplementation helps lower LDL cholesterol or "bad cholesterol", preventing serious cardiovascular diseases.
- Consumption of krill oil helps even out blood sugar levels preventing diabetes; it also helps diabetics keep their blood sugar levels in check.
- A recent study has shown that daily consumption of krill oil (300mg) helped reduce pain and stiffness in arthritis patients.
- Anecdotal evidence suggests that krill oil helps in reducing the symptoms associated with PMS (Premenstrual Syndrome).

19. Bulbine Natalensis

- An indigenous African botanical that is traditionally used in South African herbal medicine to improve potency in men
- Test results demonstrate that it helps to boost testosterone, progesterone, luteinizing hormone and follicle-stimulating hormone levels and decrease estrogen levels. Bulbine Natalensis appears to adversely affect the structure of the liver and kidneys at dosages used to increase testosterone. **Not recommended and not safe.**

BOOST TESTOSTERONE BY CONSIDERING THESE ITEMS

Buy / Use	Reasons / Effects on humans
Organic Meats and Produce	Limit toxin exposure
Natural Soaps and Shampoos	Limit toxin exposure
Use only glass containers	Limit toxin exposure

A Case for Glass Containers

There is a rather large toxic threat that we face on a daily basis and that is from plasticizers, which are a family of compounds that have been used for decades to keep plastics flexible. They are found practically in every commercial product and are everywhere. The most familiar is BPA; this persistent chemical does not break down and likes to accumulate in fat tissue. Studies have demonstrated that the levels of BPA found in the fat tissues and urine of humans where at the levels that have been found to be harmful to other species on our planet. BPA belongs to a rather large family of chemicals referred to as endocrine disruptors. Why is this a problem? The endocrine system is our bodies' communication and messaging superhighway, it is how glands talk to organs and tissue. If this messaging system gets disrupted then our crucial hormonal messages are being negatively altered.

BPA binds to the receptors on our cells that our hormones use to regulate our hormonal and physiologic functions. What BPA does is play "king of the hill" with our hormones. When BPA displaces our hormones, knocking them off their respective receptors, taking their place, BPA now sends altered cellular messages. What I find particularly disturbing is that it takes only a very small exposure to these endocrine disrupting chemicals to create changes in cellular communication and health changes.

So what can you do to get away from these endocrine disrupting chemicals? Avoid using commercially packaged foodstuffs as much as possible. Prepare your own food; use organic meats, fruits, vegetables, and nuts. When it comes to storing your foods, use glass storage containers and avoid using any plastic container, and especially do not reheat any food in a plastic container is a good way to play it safe.

Plastic recycle codes 1-7: These are the most common plastics consumers use.

Code	Name	Common Use	Recommendation
1	**PET** Polyethylene Terephthalate	Plastic bottles (soft drink, single use water bottles).	Be careful. Designed for single use only. Extended use increases risk of leaching and bacterial growth.
2	**HDPE** High density Polyethylene	Grocery bags, detergent bottles, milk and juice jugs.	Appears to be safe.
3	**PVC** Polyvinyl chloride	Garden hose, cable sheathing, window frames, blister packs.	Avoid. Nicknamed the Poison Plastic, contains many dangerous toxins.
4	**LDPE** Low density Polyethylene	Heavy duty bags, bread bags, plastic food wrap.	Appears to be safe.
5	**PP** Polypropylene	Medicine bottles, cereal liners, packing tape, straws.	Appears to be safe.
6	**PS** Polystyrene	CD & video cases, plastic cutlery, foam packaging.	Avoid. May leach styrene, a possible human carcinogen. May be a hormone disruptor.
7	**Other** **PC** Polycarbonate	Baby bottles, water cooler bottles, car parts.	Caution: Concern with leaching of Bisphenol A which appears to cause chromosomal change.

Low T Patient Profile: **Too Much Too Young**

27 year old, 5' 5", 127lb, male who works at a local pesticide company. He had a recent visit to a "commercial clinic" for Low T and was given 200mg of testosterone cypionate and now "feels bad," complains of pounding in chest, feeling anxious and wired and cannot rest.

Labs:

Glucose: 88 mg/dL
HgA1c: 5.2
Liver panel: normal
CBC: normal
PSA: 0.9
Insulin: 7.0uIU/mL
Lipid Panel: normal
Prolactin: 6.2
Cortisol AM: 19
LH: 0.1 mIU/mL
Total Testosterone: >2000ng/dL!!

Free Testosterone: 26.5pg/mL
Sensitive Estradiol: 23.0pg/mL
DHT: 78ng/dL
SHBG: 24.0nmol/L
DHEA Sulfate: 330/dL
Vitamin D: 48.2ng/mL
Serum Iron: 113ug/dL
Serum Ferritin: 195ng/mL
TSH: 1.0 uIU/mL
fT3: 3.6 pg/mL
fT4: 1.19 ng/dL

Pre-TRT Labs at commercial clinic:

Total Testosterone: 533ng/dL
Free Testosterone: 10.5pg/mL

Physical Examination revealed:

Obviously agitated demeanor
Normal blood pressure 123/76
Average testicles
DRE: unremarkable

Considerations for Differential Diagnosis:

Iatrogenic Androgen Excess
Daily Pesticide/Herbicide exposure
DHEA Deficiency
Vitamin D deficiency
Zinc deficient by Zinc Tally Test

Therapy and Recommendations:

Recover H-P-T Axis
Organophosphate detox
10-15 minute Sauna daily
Testralin two daily
Zinc 75 mg two daily
Restorative Sleep in bed by 10PM
Recommend no further testosterone delivery
10 Day Liver Detoxification along with a Mediterranean diet
Alpha Lipoic Acid daily: *α-lipoic acid (LA) is a pleiotropic compound with potential pharmacotherapeutic value against a range of pathophysiological insults.*

Omega 10 one daily
Vitamin D 5000IU Sublingual QD
DHEA 25mg twice daily
No Alcohol
No caffeine

Subjective Patient Report
Feels better and has taken another job

Follow Up Lab at 90 days:
Liver panel: normal
CBC: normal
Lipid Panel: normal
Prolactin: 6.0
Cortisol AM: 17.0
LH: 5.2 mIU/mL
Total Testosterone: 662ng/dL
Free Testosterone: 13.0pg/mL
Sensitive Estradiol: 19.6pg/mL

DHT: 42 ng/dL
SHBG: 22.0nmol/L
DHEA Sulfate: 379.0ug/dL
Vitamin D: 66.2ng/mL
Serum Iron: 145ug/dL
Serum Ferritin: 195ng/mL
SH: 1.0 uIU/mL
fT3: 3.7 pg/mL
fT4: 1.09 ng/dL

Take Home Point:
Limit your daily toxic exposure!

Chapter 7

You have Low T because you have to Heal Your Gut and Detox Your Liver

The gut contains over 100 trillion bacteria that play a vital role in our overall health. Antibiotics, stress, unhealthy foods, and toxins negatively alter these bacteria that eventually lead to a problem called dysbiosis and leaky gut. Dysbiosis is an imbalance of bacteria that can occur in any of our mucus membranes, such as in the lungs, mouth, nose, and the stomach and intestines. Dysbiosis and leaky gut are incredibly common and are initiators of inevitable illness and hormone disruption. Dysbiosis and leaky gut are often seen in people with inflammatory bowel disease, non-alcoholic fatty liver, obesity, colon cancer, IBS, diabetes, insulin resistance, leptin resistance and more. The best thing we can do for our digestive health and overall health is balance our gut bacteria.

Daily stress and toxins make us sick, tired, fat, and decrease the quality of our lives! Not only do our hormones decline with age and lose their natural rhythm, they lose their effectiveness due to the numerous toxins we are subjected to on a daily basis.

Environmental toxins contribute to metabolic disease: hypertension, abdominal fat, high cholesterol, cardiovascular disease, diabetes, and stroke. Degenerative disease: arthritis, osteoporosis, dementia, hair, vision, hearing, and muscle loss. Mental disease: anxiety, depression, ADD, bipolar, and psychosis. Toxin exposure causes allergies, asthma, eczema, psoriasis, multiple sclerosis, autoimmune and endocrine disruption, and cancer.

There are over 3800 chemicals used daily in the United States and less than half have ever been tested in humans. Over 5 million man-made chemicals have been registered in the US since 2009 alone. There are roughly 100,000 chemicals that are consumed by humans and only about 10% have been tested. The average adult when tested has about 91 different toxins in their body at any given time and umbilical cord blood sampling has found over 280 different toxins in unborn children's blood. These toxins have been linked to cancer, central nervous system disorders, hormone disruption, birth defects, and reproduction and immune system dysfunction.

Toxins

- Chemicals
- Food additives
- Household products
- Contaminants
- Drugs
- Medicines
- OTC medications
- Metabolic end products
- Bacterial toxins
- Heavy Metals
- Organophosphates

Biologically speaking our bodies are fined tuned wonders of the miracle of life. Our agile Hypothalamic-Pituitary-Thyroid/Adrenal/Gonadal Axis' communicate with target cells, glands, and organs to balance the intricate dance of our hormones creating an effective, efficient, responsive metabolic furnace. Unfortunately, age, disease, stress and toxic exposure disrupt this delicate balance leading to the acceleration of numerous disease states.

Every day we are exposed to numerous chemicals that make us feel:

- Tired
- Irritable
- Bloated
- Unhealthy
- Achy
- Moody
- Unrested
- Foggy Thinking

Your body's ability to detoxify all the harmful substances it comes in contact with is vital to your overall health and wellness. However your body's ability to adequately detox can be compromised by toxic exposure, stress, and lack of essential nutrients from poor dietary habits. Making the necessary adjustments to your lifestyle, nutrition, and toxic exposure will improve every aspect of your health. Detoxifying your body will:

- Improve your sleep
- Clearer thinking
- Improve digestion
- Enhance Mood
- More Energy
- Optimize hormones

Detoxification is a 2-step process by which the body rids itself of toxic substances. Those toxic substances can be the by-product of our own metabolism or from substances we knowingly or unknowingly have consumed. In the first step the cytochrome P450 enzyme system takes a toxin that resembles a non-soluble fat like substance and turns it into a soluble water-like substance called an intermediate. In the second step called Conjugation, conjugase enzymes take the intermediate and attach another substance to it that will allow the now water-soluble substance to be transported into the blood and excreted from the body in the urine and stool. The following nutrients aid the body in phase I and phase II liver detoxification.

DETOXIFICATION PROCESS:

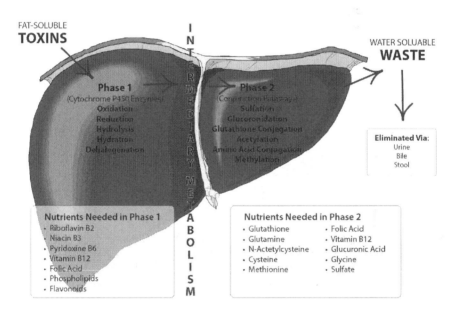

Protective Nutrients

• Copper	• Zinc	• Turmeric	• Cauliflower
• Vitamin A	• Manganese	• Green Tea	• Brussels sprouts
• Vitamin C	• Selenium	• Broccoli	• Coenzyme Q10
• Vitamin E	• Milk thistle	• Onions	• Garlic

TOXIC EXPOSURE QUIZ

1. Do you have difficulty concentrating?
2. Do you often have a lack of energy?
3. Do you feel tired all the time?
4. Do you wake up feeling sluggish?
5. Do you have heartburn or reflux?
6. Do you have digestion issues?
7. Do you have difficulty sleeping?
8. Do you have headaches?
9. Are you often irritable and moody?
10. Does your body often ache?
11. Do you work with pesticides/insecticides/chemicals?
12. Do you drink more than one or two drinks per week?
13. Do you smoke?
14. Do you eat fast food more than once per week?

If you answered yes to any of these questions then more than likely you are suffering from some degree of toxic exposure and daily detoxification of your system will improve your overall health, wellbeing, and optimize your hormones.

Steps to detoxifying your body:

- Reduce daily stress
- Sauna
- Adequate hydration with water
- Reduce/eliminate alcohol and drug use
- Healthful nutrition habits
- Appropriate supplementation
- Regular exercise that induces sweating
- Eliminate/reduce toxic exposure to metabolic waste products, antibiotics, contaminants, pollutants, insecticides, pesticides, food additives, sugar, and microorganisms

Foods to help you naturally detox

Nutrition plays a major role in the detoxification of your body. You must have adequate protein consumption to supply the necessary amino acids used by the liver to provide energy for detoxification. The most critical antioxidant and detoxifier made by the human body is glutathione. Adequate lean protein helps you make glutathione.

Healthful fruits and vegetables provide powerful phytonutrients that will help to detoxify your body. The following list is foods that will help provide the proper nutrients to allow for efficient and effective detoxification.

- Berries
- Apples
- Almonds
- Dark Chocolate
- Coffee
- Garlic
- Cilantro
- Green Tea
- Artichokes
- Pomegranate
- Brussels sprouts
- Cabbage
- Kale
- Cauliflower
- Collard greens
- Broccoli
- Broccoli sprouts – the most powerful

Every one of us is subject to stress and inflammation and to some degree. We all have to eat and it is through our intestines that our bodies intimately interact with the environment. This is why our immune system, our digestive tract is our largest immune system organ, is on constant guard with cellular defenses in our intestines. Healthy liver and healthful food choices will protect us from a leaky gut and hormone disruption.

So what exactly is a leaky gut? The lining of your digestive tract is like a "ping pong net" with extremely small holes in it that only allows specific nutrient substances to pass through it. Your intestinal lining works as a barrier keeping out bigger particles that can cause damage.

A leaky gut sometimes called increased intestinal permeability, is when the "ping pong net" in your digestive tract is damaged due to inflammation, which results in larger holes like that in a "tennis net". Now, larger substances and particles could pass through this barrier;

proteins like gluten, unfavorable bacteria, yeast, and undigested foods particles. Toxic waste can also leak from the inside of your intestinal wall into your blood stream causing further inflammation and an immune response.

Most endotoxins gain access to our intestinal circulation but they rarely ever get into our bodies to cause serious problems because our liver is there to protect our internal environment. The binding of endotoxin in the liver is increased by exercise, healthful food choices, testosterone, estrogen and even the limited use of alcohol.

An HDL > 50 is a sign of good liver function. HDL particles actually bind inflammatory endotoxin particles to increase our immunity from oxidation from many different sources. This is why a high HDL level is generally associated with health and well-being.

Cholesterol is so important to our health and the body actually makes it itself, in case we do not get enough from our diet. Our bodies make about 1000mg per day. Our bodies have the ability to regulate the amount of cholesterol in the blood, producing more when our diet doesn't provide adequate amounts. The regulation of cholesterol synthesis is a dynamic process that is integral to our overall well-being, health, and fitness.

A high HDL-P also protects us from inflammatory damage. This biologic process is one of the reasons why we see higher cholesterol levels in the face of cellular stress or infection.

The increased production of cholesterol is one of the body's natural responses if the intestinal lining is overwhelmed. We also need to be aware that any stressor can increase the permeability of the gut to endotoxic damage. This includes increased cortisol, insulin, malabsorption syndromes, grains, bacterial imbalances, poor nutrition, excess sugar or infections. The liver is assisted in its protection by the action of thyroid hormone. If your thyroid is working well, when you get intestinal inflammation, that can cause a leaky gut, your thyroid responds by increasing production of its own hormone to allow for the up-regulation of cholesterol turnover. Thyroid hormone does this by acting as a co-factor with vitamin A to allow the conversion of cholesterol to pregnenolone. Pregnenolone is the basic building block of all the steroid hormones that our brain uses to signal all the cells in our bodies. This process is also dependent upon other vitamins and minerals being in adequate supply and include; iodine, zinc, copper, selenium, Vitamins A, B3, 5,6,12, C, E, magnesium, manganese, and coenzyme Q10. I highly recommend having your intracellular nutritional status tested. Spectracell Laboratories provides such a test.

If this system is not working properly then we have a hormonal interruption between the brain and our cells. Thyroid hormones help regulate and control the inflammatory processes in our bodies. When our bodies lose control of our thyroid hormone production we essentially lose control of how the brain sends its message to our cells and we can no longer make steroid hormones effectively from pregnenolone. It explains why we see low vitamin D levels, low testosterone, low DHEA, low estrogen levels, cortisol irregularities, Na+, K-, and Ca+ issues. Rarely is a single hormone deficiency at play when there is a leaky gut involved. Pregnenolone is a steroid precursor. It is made in the body from LDL cholesterol. In order to get pregnenolone, we need adequate amounts of LDL cholesterol plus other nutrients, including vitamin A, thyroid hormone and enzymes. If any of these are inadequate, you will have a pregnenolone deficiency.

Sex Hormone Synthesis Pathways

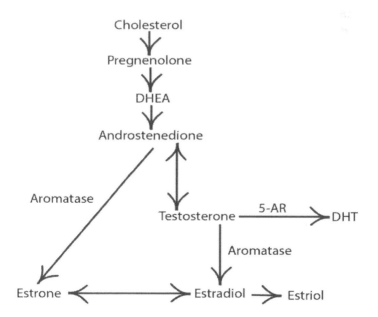

Continuing with thyroid hormone, about 20% of the conversion of T4 to T3 occurs directly in the digestive tract but outside the liver. Thyroid hormone also works to help protect our portal circulation from digestive tract inflammation. TSH is released from the anterior pituitary in the brain. In hypothyroidism, TSH is high because the pituitary is asking the thyroid gland to make more active thyroid hormone or T4. T4 has to be converted to the active form of thyroid hormone called T3. The remainder of this conversion is in the liver, about 80%. So you now see the connection between the production of hormones, which starts in the brain, the digestive tract that is our first line of defense against inflammation, and the liver which helps to detoxify our internal environment and is responsible for the production of energy and the initial steps in the manufacturing of many essential hormones.

This inflammatory state started in the gut, spread to the liver and to the rest of the body, also causes the liver to make high sensitivity-CRP. High sensitivity-CRP or cardiac-CRP is what we used to measure inflammation in the body. It is called an acute phase reactant protein. High CRP levels are associated with inflammation in the lining of the blood vessels, called the endothelium. Inflammation of the endothelium is one factor which leads to the development of atherosclerosis. The increased CRP demonstrates that there are numerous pro inflammatory chemicals like cytokines throughout the body. Inflammatory cytokines released in the inflammatory process suppress the production of thyrotropoin releasing hormone, TRH, thyroid stimulating hormone, TSH, reduce the production of T4, and reduce the conversion of T4 to T3, and lead to the increase of reverse T3. In short, the more inflammation you have the less active thyroid hormone is available for all the cells and tissues throughout the body. Inflammation caused by infection, obesity, diabetes, pre-diabetes or insulin resistance, autoimmune disease, poor nutrition, alcohol abuse, substance abuse, and smoking all contribute to the overall derangement of multiple hormone synthesis pathways.

So as you can see elevated TSH levels with low free T3 levels and elevated reverse T3 are not good signs. An underactive thyroid, subclinical hypothyroidism, or overt hypothyroidism is correlated with heart disease and many autoimmune conditions. Hashimoto's thyroiditis is at epidemic proportions in the United States and is indicative intestinal inflammation that eventually overwhelms the portal circulation and liver with inflammation that then spreads throughout the entire body.

This results in a response from the liver where a once favorable Pattern A LDL 1+2 with a high HDL2 changes to unfavorable Pattern B LDL 4+3 with a low HDL2, a high HDL3, and a high HS-CRP. Now, the body is staged for an inevitable life-threatening, potentially catastrophic event, like a heart attack. As you can see there is more at risk here than just low-T.

Once the inflammation is present in the circulation it precedes to the two most prominent organs based upon blood flow, the brain and the heart. In the brain the first effect is to overwhelm the parts that are not protected by the brain blood barrier. The most important are the hypothalamus and pituitary glands, where TRH and TSH are made, respectively. This is another way the thyroid gland's production of T4 can be decreased resulting in the decrease conversion of T4 to T3 and causes a problem with the conversion of cholesterol to pregnenolone. Remember, we need active T3 to convert LDL cholesterol to pregnenolone. The disruption of this complex cascade results in the breakdown of cellular homeostasis leading to disease development. In the heart the hs-CRP encourages the development of atheroma generation in the coronary arteries and stiffens the leaflets of the heart valves. It also causes changes to the heart's electrical system leading to heart arrhythmias. As the atheroma collects OxLDL, oxidized LDL, in combination with elevated HS-CRP the plaque eventually ruptures and causes a heart attack or even worse, death.

My go to statin when medically necessary is rosuvastatin.

The Jupiter Study showed that rosuvastatin (Crestor) lowers cardiac-CRP by 37%, LDL by 50% with a 60% decrease in heart attacks and sudden death and a 70% reduction in stroke. Statins do increase the incidence of diabetes; however the prevention of cardiovascular disease outweighs the risk of diabetes.

My Go To Supplements To Improve Cholesterol Profile:

- Omega 10
- Berberine
- Vitamin C
- Policosanol
- Red Yeast Rice
- Niatain

Now you can see how the brain, the digestive tract, and liver are intimately connected and important to our overall health. Our digestive tract is our first line of defense, the liver is the last line of defense before the brain and our hormones are affected. Once the brain is assaulted hormonal disruption occurs and the brain loses control over hormonal homeostasis. We can understand this entire process when we take a closer look at our NMR Lipid Profile. The NMR Lipid Profile provides a direct measurement of lipids and other risk factors for cardiovascular disease. In my opinion this test informs us of the overall insult on our brain, liver, digestive tract, and ultimately our hormones and is perhaps the single most valuable test your doctor may have never even heard of and the one you want done today.

Understanding an NMR LipoProfile Test Result

Understanding the Science

Scientists know that heart disease is partly caused by particles in the blood called low-density lipoproteins, or LDL. But without the tools to measure these LDL particles directly, physicians have historically calculated their numbers by measuring the cholesterol they contain. This measure is known as LDL cholesterol, or LDL-C.

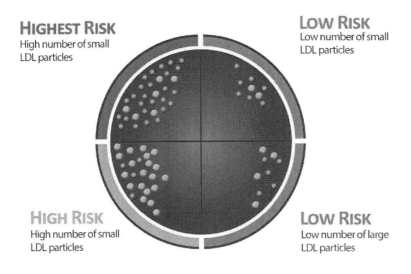

HIGHEST RISK
High number of small LDL particles

LOW RISK
Low number of small LDL particles

HIGH RISK
High number of small LDL particles

LOW RISK
Low number of large LDL particles

While useful for some patients, knowing the amount of cholesterol in these particles is not as important as knowing the actual number of LDL particles. When high numbers of LDL particles are in the blood, they build up in the arteries and cause heart disease. So a higher number of LDL particles (LDL-P) indicate a higher risk of heart disease.

Your LDL-P Number

The LDL-P number is the most crucial part of the NMR LipoProfile report. The lower this number is, the less risk for cardiovascular disease. In the sample diagram below, the relative risk of the LDL-P score is indicated by the highlighted box. The higher the LDL-P number is, the boxes further to the right will be highlighted. The lower the number, the highlighted box will shift to the left.

The LDL-P number can range from less than 1000 to more than 2000. Based on this number, your physician can recommend a treatment plan designed to lower your risk level. The LDL-P goal will depend on your particular medical history.

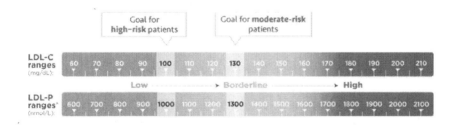

Small LDL-P Number

The Small LDL-P is a measure of the number of small LDL particles in the blood. These particles are associated with an increased risk of heart disease; more of these small particles lead to greater risk for cardiovascular disease. The Small LDL particle score can vary widely, with a lower score being much better. Individuals are generally at lower risk for heart disease if their Small LDL-P is less than 700. Individuals are at the lowest risk when both their LDL-P and Small LDL-P number are low. Your doctor will look at both these numbers to determine your heart disease risk and to develop a treatment plan if necessary.

Treatment Options

If test results show an increased risk for heart disease, then your doctor can discuss various options with you to lower your risk. These options include lifestyle adjustments, such as increased exercise and changes in nutrition. In some cases your doctor may recommend supplements or prescription medications, which may be effective in lowering your LDL-P and Small LDL-P numbers.

Your physician may choose from these commonly prescribed medications to lower your LDL-P and Small LDL-P numbers.

So how do we heal that Leaky Gut?

Digestive Dysfunction-Leaky Gut-Increased Intestinal Permeability

Leaky Gut is the result of damage to the intestinal lining that makes it less able to protect the internal environment as well as to absorb needed nutrients and other biological substances. Consequently, bacteria and their toxins, incompletely digested proteins and fats, and waste not normally absorbed may "leak" out of the intestines into the blood stream. This triggers an autoimmune reaction, which can lead to gastrointestinal problems such as bloating, excessive gas and cramps, fatigue, numerous food sensitivities, achy joints, rashes, and hormonal imbalances. The cause of this syndrome may be chronic inflammation from toxic exposure, food sensitivities, chronic stress, damage from taking large amounts of medications, cytotoxic drugs and radiation or antibiotics, excessive alcohol consumption, or a compromised immune system and our pro-inflammatory modern food sources, especially wheat.

Causes of Leaky Gut:

- Poor Nutrition: refined sugars, processed foods, preservatives, and refined flours
- Chronic Stress: comes in various forms
- Inflammation: hypoacidity of the stomach & inflammation of any type
- Medications: acetaminophen, aspirin, and antibiotics
- Zinc deficiency
- Candida overgrowth

Leaky gut Results in:

- Malabsorption of vitamins
- Malabsorption of minerals especially iron and zinc
- Low thyroid hormone
- Decreased steroid hormone synthesis

Stop Your Leaky Gut

- Avoid Alcohol
- Avoid nonsteroidal anti-inflammatory drugs
- Avoid antibiotics
- Limit Caffeine
- Eliminate conventional dairy
- Eliminate genetically modified foods
- Eliminate all processed sugars
- Avoid whole grains
- Add Omega 3/Omega 7
- Follow a low glycemic nutrition plan/Paleo plan
- Repair intestinal lining
- Restore pancreatic enzymes
- Inoculate the digestive tract with beneficial bacteria
- Replace fiber in your diet

On the following page are a series of questions related to specific areas of your digestive system. In each section assess how you have been feeling over the previous 3 months. If you have experienced any or all of these symptoms at least 2-3 times per week answer "yes". If you answer yes to 3 or more of these questions in each section, then you are experiencing problems related to that specific area of your digestive tract. If the above suggestions of elimination are only partially successful or unsuccessful you may need some of the suggested supplements listed below. You can find these supplements by Metagenics ® at our online store. www.alphamaleinstitute.com/the-alpha-male-store/

Gastric Function Questions

1. Do you have indigestion?
2. Do you have excessive belching, burping, or bloating after meals?
3. Do you have stomach spasms or cramping after you eat?
4. Do you have a feeling of pressure like food is just sitting in your stomach?
5. Do you have a bad taste in your mouth after you eat?
6. Does a small amount of food fill you up?
7. Do you skip meals or eat erratically because you are not hungry?

If you answered yes to 3 or more of these questions in this section, then you are experiencing problems related to gastric hypoacidity. The following Metagenics ® supplements may help alleviate your symptoms.

Ultraflora Balance: one twice daily
Endefen: two tablespoons daily
Metagest: one three times daily
Zinlori: Two tablets daily

Gastric Inflammation Questions

1. Does the thought of or smell of food aggravate your stomach?
2. Do you feel hungry an hour or two after eating a meal?
3. Do you have stomach pain an hour or two after eating?
4. Do you have stomach pain relieved by eating food or drinking milk or taking antacids?
5. Do you have a burning sensation in the lower part of your chest especially if you lie down?
6. Do you have digestive issue that gets better with rest?
7. Does eating spicy food, fatty food, coffee, alcohol, or hot peppers cause your stomach to burn?
8. Do you have difficulty swallowing food or liquids?

If you answer yes to 3 or more of these questions in this section, then you are experiencing problems related to gastric inflammation. The following Metagenics ® supplements may help alleviate your symptoms.

Ultraflora Balance: one twice daily
Endefen: two tablespoons daily
GI Sustain: 2 scoops in 8oz. of water twice daily

Pancreas and Small Intestine Questions

1. Is there pain to the touch under your rib cage on the left side?
2. Do you have delayed indigestion for 2-4 hours after you eat?
3. Do you have lower abdominal pain that is relieved by passing gas of having a bowel movement?
4. Do you have specific foods that aggravate your indigestion regularly?
5. Does the consistency of your stools change daily?
6. Is your stool odor strong?
7. Do you have undigested food in your stool?
8. Do you have 3 or more bowel movements a day?
9. Do you have frequent diarrhea?
10. Do you have a bowel movement immediately after you eat?

If you answered yes to 3 or more of these questions in this section, then you are experiencing problems related to digestive enzymes. The following Metagenics ® supplements may help alleviate your symptoms.

Ultraflora Balance: one twice daily
Endefen: two tablespoons daily
Azeo-Pangen: one three times daily
SpectraZyme: 2 tablets daily

Colon Questions

1. Do you have pain or cramps in your lower abdominal region?
2. Do raw fruits and vegetables cause abdominal pain and bloating?
3. Are you often constipated?
4. Is your stool hard, small, and pebble like?
5. Do you pass mucus in your stool?
6. Do you have days of constipation and days with diarrhea?
7. Do you have rectal pain, itching, or cramping?
8. Days where you have no urge to have a bowel movement?
9. Almost a constant need to have a bowel movement?

If you answered yes to 3 or more of these questions in this section, then you are experiencing problems related to the colon. The following Metagenics ® supplements may help alleviate your symptoms.

Ultraflora Balance: one twice daily
Endefen: two tablespoons daily
Herbulk: one scoop in 8oz. of water daily
Glutagenics: one teaspoon with water three times daily

Liver and Gallbladder Questions

1. If you massage under your rib cage on the right, is it tender or painful?
2. Do you have abdominal pain that worsens with deep breathing?
3. Do you have right-sided abdominal pain that moves to your back or right shoulder?
4. Anything bitter gives you indigestion?
5. Do you have abdominal pain, nausea, or indigestion from eating fatty or fried foods?
6. Do you get headaches if you overeat?
7. Do you have itchy skin at night that is not dry?
8. Does your stool change colors from light brown to a white-clay color?
9. Do you feel lethargic and in poor health?
10. Do your muscles ache even though you have not exercised?
11. Are you often swollen in the abdomen?
12. Do you have a funny body odor?
13. Do you often have bad breath?
14. Do you bruise easily?
15. Do the whites of your eyes have a yellowish tinge to them?

If you answer yes to 3 or more of these questions in this section, then you are experiencing problems related to hepatobiliary function. The following Metagenics ® supplements may help alleviate your symptoms.

Ultraflora Balance: one twice daily
Endefen: two tablespoons daily
Lipo-Gen: one tablet three times daily

Suggested Metagenics® Products:

Available only through a licensed physician, the line of products from Metagenics provides a level of quality high above other supplements on the market. All of the supplements listed in this chapter are available in our store at www.alphamaleinstitute.com/the-alpha-male-store/

* These statements have not been evaluated by the Food and Drug Administration. These products are not intended to diagnose, treat, cure, or prevent any disease.

Azeo-Pangen: one three times daily

Azeo-Pangen™ is a comprehensive enzyme complex that provides support for healthy digestive function. * The porcine pancreatic concentrate is processed under special conditions so that the delicate enzyme constituents remain intact.

Endefen: two tablespoons daily

Endefen™ is uniquely designed to nutritionally support the health and function of the gastrointestinal (GI) tract. This exceptional formula addresses multiple factors that contribute to GI health.
- Supports the integrity of the gastric lining by promoting the growth of gastric mucosal cells.
- Provides lecithin and astaxanthin, which have demonstrated protective effects on the gastric environment.
- Provides arabinogalactans and green tea, which may help promote the growth of healthy intestinal microflora.
- Arabinogalactans may help promote the production of beneficial short-chain fatty acids, an important fuel for intestinal cells.
- Provides plantain, which has been shown in a lab to support the integrity of the gastric lining.
- Provides targeted antioxidants to help protect the gastric mucosa.
- Provides key nutrients to enhance GI immune system function.

GI Sustain: 2 scoops in 8oz. of water twice daily

GI Sustain™ is a medical food formulated to provide specialized nutritional support, including amino acids and prebiotic fiber, combined with readily digestible, low-allergenic-potential macronutrients for patients with leaky gut syndrome. Featuring L-glutamine and isomalto-oligosaccharides (IMO), this formula supports intestinal mucosal integrity and promotes the growth of beneficial bacteria to address dysbiosis associated with leaky gut syndrome.

- Supports microbial balance.
- Nourishes the cells of the colonic mucosa.
- Features low-allergy-potential rice protein concentrate supplemented with L-lysine HCl and L-threonine for an improved protein source.
- Provides rice syrup solids as a natural energy source.
- Provides a readily absorbed and metabolized lipid source.
- Provides the prebiotic IMO to selectively nourish beneficial bacteria, including lactobacillus and bifidobacteria.
- IMO is a gentle fiber that is naturally sweet but has a low-glycemic index.
- Formulated with nutrients such as zinc gluconate and L-glutamine to nutritionally support gastrointestinal mucosa integrity.
- Supports microbial balance.
- Nourishes the cells of the colonic mucosa.
- Features low-allergy-potential rice protein concentrate supplemented with L-lysine HCl and L-threonine for an improved protein source.
- Provides rice syrup solids as a natural energy source.
- Provides a readily absorbed and metabolized lipid source.
- Provides the prebiotic IMO to selectively nourish beneficial bacteria, including lactobacillus and bifidobacteria.
- IMO is a gentle fiber that is naturally sweet but has a low-glycemic index.
- Formulated with nutrients such as zinc gluconate and L-glutamine to nutritionally support gastrointestinal mucosa integrity.

Glutagenics: one teaspoon with water three times daily

Glutagenics® features three key ingredients--glutamine, deglycyrrhizinized licorice (DGL), and aloe--that are designed to support the integrity and healthy function of the gastrointestinal lining. A healthy gastrointestinal lining is essential for proper digestion, immune function, and overall health. Glutagenics supplies:

- 3.5 grams of the amino acid glutamine, which provides both a source of fuel and precursors for growth to the rapidly dividing cells of the intestinal lining.
- A concentrated extract of DGL to support gastrointestinal health.
- A premium extract of aloe leaf containing polysaccharides to support a healthy intestinal lining.
- Natural flavors for improved taste.
- The licorice in Glutagenics has been processed to remove glycyrrhizin, which has been associated with sodium and water retention. In addition, a proprietary extraction process removes the bitter principles of aloe to prevent a laxative effect.
- Supports a healthy intestinal lining, which is essential for healthy digestion, healthy immune function, and overall health.
- Supplies high levels of the amino acid glutamine, which provides both a source of fuel and precursors for growth to the rapidly dividing cells of the intestinal lining.
- Provides a concentrated licorice extract that has been processed to remove glycyrrhizin, reducing the risk of adverse effects associated with licorice.
- The processing and removal of the bitter principles in aloe prevent a laxative effect.*
- Powdered form for ease of use and flexible dosing.

Herbulk: one scoop in 8oz. of water daily

Herbulk® features 7 grams of dietary fiber per serving. This low-sodium, powdered formula is designed to support healthy intestinal function and integrity, and offers great support for those occasional loose stools.

- Supports healthy intestinal function.
- Great for those who have occasional loose stools.
- Supplies satiety-enhancing fiber to create a feeling of fullness.

Lipo-Gen: one tablet three times daily

Lipo-Gen™ is a highly specialized formula that features a unique blend of lipotropic nutrients combined with select amino acids, vitamins , and a proprietary extract of herbs to support healthy liver and gallbladder function.*

- Provides nutrients involved in fat metabolism, including inositol, choline, and taurine.*
- Delivers methyl donors, folic acid, vitamins B6 and B12, and select herbs that are traditionally used to support bile flow and healthy liver function.

Metagest: one three times daily

Metagest® features betaine HCl combined with pepsin—a proteolytic enzyme—to complement the natural production of digestive agents in the stomach.

- Provides betaine HCl and pepsin, which support the breakdown of food in the stomach.
- Complements the natural production of digestive agents that may decrease as a result of environmental, dietary, or age-related factors.

Ultraflora Balance: one twice daily

UltraFlora™ Balance provides a dairy-free base for a proprietary blend of highly viable, pure strains of *L. acidophilus* NCFM® and *B. lactis* Bi-07— "friendly" bacteria that have been shown to support a healthy intestinal environment and immune health. Backed by the Metagenics ID Guarantee for purity, clinical reliability, and predicted safety via scientific identification of strains with established health benefits.

- Daily support for GI and immune health.
- Helps maintain a healthy balance of intestinal flora.
- Facilitates the digestion of lactose

UltrInflamX Plus 360: 2 scoops in 8oz. of water daily

UltraInflamX® PLUS 360° is a medical food formulated to provide specialized nutritional support for patients with compromised gut function reflective of an inflammatory response as seen in ulcerative colitis and Crohn's disease. Provided in a low-allergenic-potential rice protein base, this formula is enhanced with antioxidant nutrients, selenium, zinc, calcium, folate, and vitamin B12 to address increased nutrient needs and potential deficiencies in these patients. L-glutamine is added to support intestinal mucosal cells. This formula is acceptable for an enteral diet that excludes allergens. Enteral and exclusion diets are often necessary for extended periods for patients experiencing irritable bowel conditions.

Zinlori: Two tablets daily

Zinlori 75™ contains a high potency, zinc-carnosine complex formulated to provide relief of stomach discomfort. Zinc-carnosine works by supporting the healthy ecology, natural defenses, and integrity of the stomach lining. Zinc-carnosine is a well-researched natural supplement for gastric discomfort.
- Supports a healthy gastric environment.
- Helps relieve mild and occasional gastric discomforts, including heartburn, nausea, bloating, and upset stomach.
- Promotes a healthy gastric microbial balance.
- Helps maintain the integrity of the protective gastric mucosal lining possibly by supporting healthy mucus secretion.
- Some research indicates that zinc-carnosine may protect gastric mucosal cells without altering prostaglandin metabolism.
- Gastro-supportive benefits demonstrated in over 20 published studies.
- Same raw material used successfully by healthcare practitioners in Japan since 1994.
- Does not affect stomach digestion.

Consider the New Super Food Hiding in your Grocery Store

Broccoli Sprouts

Part of the cellular defense mechanism is the production of antioxidant compounds to quench Reactive Oxygen Species or Oxidants. Part of the cell's internal defense mechanism is the Nrf2-ARE pathway (*nuclear erythroid 2 related factor 2 -antioxidant responsive element)*, which up regulates many protective detoxification and antioxidant genes acting synergistically to increase the efficacy of cellular defense. The Nrf2-ARE pathway is the master regulator of cytoprotective genes and activates over 500 cytoprotective genes. This pathway may also be the master regulator of the aging process as well.

Nrf2 activation increases the expression of genes coding for these important cellular defenses:

- Glutithione-the major intracellular antioxidant
- Vitamin D receptors
- BRCA1 and BRCA2
- Ferritin-binds free iron
- Quinone reductase- detoxifies estrogen
- Metallothionein-binds heavy metals
- Gluathione-S-transferase- an essential detoxifying enzyme

There is strong evidence that increased expression of the Nrf2-ARE regulated genes inhibits cancer development.

(Zhang Y et al. A Strategy for Cancer Prevention: Stimulation of the Nrf2-ARE signaling pathway. Mol Cancer Therapy 2004; 3(7) July

Sulforaphane is the most potent phytochemical activator of Nrf2. Where do we find this potent activator of cellular defense? Broccoli Sprouts!

Why the Sprout vs. the mature vegetable?

Glucoraphanin in sprouts is the precursor to Sulforaphane and is 20-50 times greater than in mature broccoli.

Sulforaphane is formed when the myrosinase and glucoraphanin inside the broccoli sprout vacuole are ruptured by chewing.

**Broccoli sprout or seed extracts do not contain myrosinase and provides no clinical effect!!!

So if you are looking to turn on cancer protective genes and detoxify your body start eating your broccoli sprouts!

When I walk into the fruit and vegetable section of the grocery store I see healing, powerful, cancer protective, energy giving nutrients capable of curing many of today's lifestyle diseases and you should too. Eating healthful is taking command of your personal health and fitness and speaks to your body on a molecular level empowering your full genetic potential.

Chapter 8

Check Your Nutrition

Whether you have a consistent, healthful dietary plan or you are a regular consumer of the typical American diet of heavily processed foods, salt, sugar, toxins, soda, and hormones. You very may well be nutritionally deficient in numerous vitamins and minerals. Most of our foods are completely lacking the necessary vitamins, minerals and healthful fats essential for creating optimal human bodily functioning and raising your testosterone.

Almost nearly all the necessary vitamins, minerals, antioxidants and fiber that we need come from the fruits and vegetables that we eat on a regular basis. Healthy diets rich in fruits and vegetables may reduce the risk of cancer, chronic disease and low testosterone. It has been my personal experience and in working with our patients that diets rich in dark leafy green vegetables and low sugar fruits improve and reverse lifestyle diseases such as hypertension, high cholesterol, insulin resistance, diabetes, obesity, and inflammatory diseases which decreases ones chances for serious medical consequences such as heart attacks, stroke, early death, and poor quality of life.

The nutritional quizzes on the following pages I have outlined for you will help disclose if you have any deficiencies in these important vitamins, minerals, and fats that help drive numerous metabolic functions. If you answer yes to 3 or more questions in each section, you may have a deficiency with that particular nutrient. Optimizing their levels will help you to improve your personal health profile. While this questionnaire will help identify deficiencies, having an intracellular nutrient test performed will identify your exact deficiencies. You can get one of these tests performed at SpectraCell Laboratory.

The following intracellular nutrient test of this patient disclosed a significant deficiency in both calcium and zinc and borderline deficiencies in other vitamins and minerals. This kind of precision testing allows for personalized supplementation with the greatest benefit, which ultimately can increase testosterone to desirable levels.

The SpectraCell report below shows the different levels of nutrients in a patient along with markers to show the ranges from adequate to deficient.

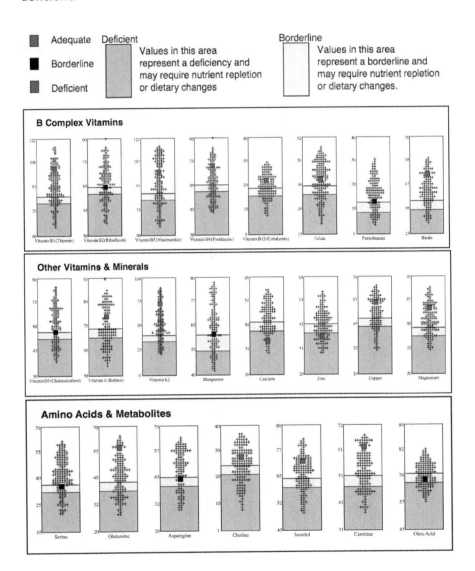

Magnesium

	Yes	No
I have a low intake of dark green leafy vegetables.		
I am tired all the time.		
I have trouble falling asleep or have insomnia.		
I have acid reflux often.		
I have difficult bowel movements.		
I have asthma.		
I experience leg or hand cramps.		
I experience muscle twitching.		
I frequently experience headaches or migraines.		
I have premenstrual syndrome most months.		
Swallowing is sometimes difficult.		
I have restless leg syndrome.		
I am sensitive to loud noises.		
I am irritable or get annoyed easily.		
I am depressed.		
I am anxious.		
I have attention deficit disorder.		
I have a lot of stress in my life.		
I have kidney stones.		
I experience heart flutters, skipped beats, or palpitations.		
I have heart disease or heart failure.		
I have mitral valve prolapse.		
I have diabetes.		
TOTAL		

Vitamin D

	Yes	No
I work indoors.		
I hardly ever go out in the sun.		
I wear sun block most of the time.		
I have seasonal affective disorder (SAD) or the winter blues.		
I have dark skin.		
I am sixty years old or older.		
I don't eat small fatty fish such as mackerel, herring, or sardines.		
My muscles are sore or weak.		
My bones are tender. (Press on your shin bone-if it hurts, you are vitamin D deficient).		
I have osteoarthritis. (Vitamin D deficiency weakens bones and leads to deterioration.)		
I have osteoporosis.		
I have broken more than two bones or fractured a hip.		
My mental sharpness and/or memory are not what they used to be.		
I have an autoimmune disease (e.g., multiple sclerosis).		
I seem to have more infections than most people I know.		
TOTAL		

Omega-3 Fatty Acids

	Yes	No
My skin is dry, itchy, scaling, or flaking.		
My nails are soft, cracked, or brittle.		
I have dandruff.		
I have hard earwax.		
I have tiny bumps on the backs of my arms or on my trunk.		
I am thirsty most of the time.		
My joints feel achy or stiff.		
I have difficult bowel movements.		
My stool is light-colored, hard, or foul-smelling.		
I am depressed, have ADD/ADHD, and/or memory loss.		
I suffer from premenstrual syndrome. (PMS)		
My blood pressure is higher than it should be.		
My LDL cholesterol it too high, my HDL cholesterol is too low, and my triglycerides are high.		
TOTAL		

Thyroid

	Yes	No
The outer thirds of my eyebrows are thinning.		
I am sensitive to cold.		
My hands and feet are cold all the time.		
My hair is thinning and/or falling out.		
I have thick skin and fingernails.		
My skin is dry.		
I experience muscle fatigue, pain or weakness.		
I have heavy menstrual bleeding, serious PMS, other menstrual problems, or infertility.		
My sex drive has decreased.		
I am tired all the time, especially in the morning.		
My memory and concentration are not what they used to be.		
I have swollen feet and hands.		
I have difficulty losing weight or have recently gained weight.		
I am frequently constipated.		
I am depressed and apathetic.		
I have an autoimmune disease (e.g., rheumatoid arthritis, multiple sclerosis, lupus, allergies, or yeast overgrowth).		
I have low blood pressure and a low heart rate.		
I am gluten-sensitive or have celiac disease.		
I have been exposed to environmental toxins.		
I consume a lot of ocean fish or I have multiple dental silver (mercury) fillings.		
I have been exposed to radiation treatments.		
Thyroid problems run in my family		
TOTAL		

Sex Hormone Imbalance

For Women	Yes	No
I have irregular cycles, heave bleeding, or light bleeding.		
Prior to my period, I often get headaches and/or migraines.		
My breasts are tender and enlarged.		
I frequently have PMS.		
I am experiencing peri- or menopausal symptoms.		
I have hot flashes.		
I no longer have any interest in sex.		
I have dry skin, hair, and/or vagina.		
I experience monthly with fluctuation.		
I have gained weight around the middle.		
I feel bloated most of the time.		
I experience edema, swelling, puffiness, or water retention.		
I get premenstrual cravings (especially for sweet or salty food).		
I have frequent mood swings.		
I feel anxious.		
I am depressed.		
I feel unable to cope with ordinary demands.		
I have back, joint. or muscle pain.		
I suffer from infertility.		
I use birth control pills or other hormones		
I have breast cysts to lumps, or fibrocystic breasts.		
Breast, ovarian, or uterine cancer runs in my family.		
I have uterine fibroids.		
I have night sweats.		
I have trouble sleeping.		
I sometime have heart palpitations.		
My memory and concentration are not what they used to be.		
I have facial hair.		
I have been exposed to pesticides or heavy metals 9 in food, water, and/or the air),		
TOTAL		

Sex Hormone Imbalance

For Men	Yes	No
I have "man boobs" or have lost hair on my arms, legs, and chest.		
I am often tired or have low energy.		
I feel a sense of apathy toward my life and future.		
I have lost my vitality and sex drive.		
I have trouble achieving or maintaining an erection.		
I am infertile or have low sperm counts.		
I have loss of muscle.		
I have increased abdominal fat.		
I feel weak.		
I have bone loss or bone fractures.		
My cholesterol levels have increased.		
My insulin and blood sugar levels have increased.		
I am suffering from depression.		
I have been exposed to pesticides or heavy metals (in food, water, and/or the air.		
TOTAL		

Infections

	Yes	No
I frequently get colds and infections.		
I have recurring sinusitis.		
I have seasonal or environmental allergies.		
I have a history of chronic infections, such as hepatitis, skin infections, canker sores, cold sores.		
I have food allergies or sensitivities, or I don't feel well after eating (sluggishness, headaches, confusion, etc.),		
My work environment includes poor lighting, chemicals, and/or poor ventilation.		
I have had a heart attack or have heart disease.		
I have diabetes or am overweight (BMI greater than 25).		
I have bronchitis or asthma.		
I have eczema, acne, and/or rashes.		
I have arthritis (osteoarthritis/degenerative).		
I have an autoimmune disease (rheumatoid arthritis, lupus, hypothyroidism, etc.).		
I suffer from colitis or inflammatory bowel disease.		
I have irritable bowel syndrome (spastic colon).		
I have neuritis (ADHD, autism, mood, and behavior problems).		
Parkinson's or Alzheimer's disease runs in my family.		
My life is very stressful.		
I drink more than three alcoholic beverages a week.		
I don't exercise more than 30 minutes three time a week.		
At work, I am exposed to pesticides, toxic chemical, loud noise, heavy metals, and/or toxic bosses and coworkers.		
TOTAL		

Digestion

	Yes	No
I get heartburn		
I regularly use antacids (Tums, Maalox, acid-blocking drugs, etc.).		
I feel bloated or full, and/or have belching, burning, or flatulence, right after meals.		
Eating bread or other sugars causes bloating.		
I have chronic yeast or fungal infections (jock itch, vaginal yeast infection, athlete's foot, toenail fungus).		
I have chronic abdominal pain.		
I feel fatigued after eating.		
I often experience diarrhea.		
I have a bowel movement less than once or twice a day.		
My stools are greasy, large, poorly formed, or foul-smelling.		
I sometimes notice food that is not fully digested in my stool		
I have food allergies, intolerance, or reactions.		
I have thrush (whitish tongue).		
I have bleeding gums or gingivitis.		
I have a map-like rash on my tongue indication food allergy or yeast overgrowth.		
I have sores on my tongue.		
I frequently get canker sores.		
I drink more than three alcoholic beverages a week.		
I crave sweets and bread.		
My life is excessively stressful.		
I have a history of NSAID (ibuprofen, naproxen, etc.) or other anti-inflammatory use.		
TOTAL		

Energy Metabolism

	Yes	No
I am experiencing chronic or prolonged fatigue.		
I'm too tired to do many of the things I would like to do.		
Fatigue interferes with my work, family, or social life.		
I am not refreshed when I wake up.		
I have trouble falling or staying asleep, or I wake up too early.		
I have aching muscle pain or discomfort.		
I have muscle weakness.		
I have a poor tolerance for exercise and I'm incredibly tired afterward.		
My concentration and memory are not what they used to be.		
I am irritable and moody.		
I gained weight and developed diabetes after an acute stressor, infection, or trauma.		
I frequently overeat.		
I have been exposed to pesticides, unfiltered water, nonorganic food or other environmental chemicals.		
I have chronic fatigue syndrome or fibromyalgia.		
I have a history of chronic infections.		
I have been under prolonged stress.		
I have Gulf War syndrome.		
I have a neurologic disease (Alzheimer's, Parkinson's ALS, etc.).		
I have autism or ADHD.		
I suffer from depression, bipolar disease or schizrenia.		
TOTAL		

Oxidative Stress or Rusting

	Yes	No
Exercise is not a part of my regular routine, or is too much a part of my regular routine (more than 15 hour a week).		
I am overweight (BMI more than 25).		
I am fatigued on a regular basis.		
I sleep less than eight hours a night.		
I regularly experience deep muscle or joint pain.		
I am sensitive to perfume, smoke, or other chemicals or fumes.		
I am exposed to a significant level of environmental toxins (pollutants, chemicals, etc.) at home and/or at work.		
I drink more than three alcoholic beverages a week.		
I smoke cigarettes or cigars (or anything else).		
There is a significant amount of secondhand smoke where I work or live.		
I don't use sun block, I like to bake in the sun, or I go to tanning booths.		
I would rate my life as very stressful.		
I eat fewer than five servings of deeply colored vegetable and fruits a day.		
M diet includes a fair amount of fried foods, margarine, or a lot of animal fat (meat, cheese, etc.).		
I eat white flour and sugar more than twice a week.		
I suffer from chronic colds and infections (cold sores, canker sores, etc.).		
I don't take antioxidants or a multivitamin.		
I take prescription, over-the-counter, and/or recreational drugs.		
I have arthritis or allergies.		
I have diabetes or heart disease.		
TOTAL		

Stress and Adrenal Fatigue

	Yes	No
My life is very stressful.		
I am easily startled and suffer from panic attacks.		
I feel tired but wired.		
When I'm nervous, my palms and feet get sweaty.		
I feel fatigued.		
I often feel weak and shaky.		
When I stand up, I feel dizzy.		
I have dark circles under my eyes.		
I crave sweets.		
I crave salt.		
I don't feel refreshed after a night's sleep.		
I have difficulty either falling or staying asleep.		
I have trouble concentrating or suffer from mental fogginess.		
I frequently experience headaches.		
I catch colds easily and suffer from frequent infections.		
I can't start my day without caffeine.		
I retain water.		
I experience heart palpitations.		
I have poor tolerance for alcohol, caffeine, and other drugs.		
I don't tolerate exercise well and I'm incredibly tired afterward.		
I have hypoglycemia (low blood sugar).		
My muscles are weak.		
My blood pressure is low.		
TOTAL		

Low T Patient Profile: **Watch out for Genetics**

Michael - Age 42: VP of IT

42-year-old, 5' 8", 180lb, professional male complains of worsening erectile dysfunction, loss of libido, muscle tenderness especially after exercise, brain fog, and constant abdominal complaints especially after eating sometimes accompanied with worsening brain fog and headache. "Sometimes the world just "feels" grey." "No matter what I do, I just don't feel like myself anymore."

DXA: Excellent bone mineralization, body composition 13% free fat mass
VO2: Excellent results
Neurocognitive evaluation: Decreased executive function and verbal memory
Carotid Ultrasound with CIMT: No signs of plaque or thickening
VENDYS Testing: Decreased endothelial function

Labs:

Glucose: 90mg/dL
HgA1c: 5.1
Liver panel: normal
CBC: normal
PSA: 0.9
Insulin: 6.0uIU/mL
Lipid Panel: normal
Prolactin: 5.3
Cortisol AM: 18
LH: 5.6 mIU/mL
Total Testosterone: 633ng/dL

Free Testosterone: 12.2pg/mL
Sensitive Estradiol: 13.0pg/mL
DHT: 66ng/dL
SHBG: 64.0nmol/L!
DHEA Sulfate: 330/dL
Vitamin D: 30.2ng/mL
Serum Iron: 123ug/dL
Serum Ferritin: 155ng/mL
TSH: 1.2 uIU/mL
fT3: 3.4 pg/mL
fT4: 1.19 ng/dL

Physical Examination revealed:

Normal blood pressure 122/74
Average testicles
DRE: unremarkable
Obviously aggravated and frustrated appearance, but well-nourished with good muscle structure

Dietary History:

Investigation of dietary habits revealed extended period of calorie restriction (extended calorie restriction will elevate SHBG) with foods high in sulfates/sulfites! AH HA! In office urinary sulfites > 1600!

Sulfites are Neurotoxic!

Considerations for Differential Diagnosis:

Androgen Deficiency
Excessive SHBG due to calorie restriction
Vitamin D deficiency
Zinc deficient by Zinc Tally Test
Gastric Inflammation
Methylation Defect

Initial Therapy and Recommendations:

- 10 Day Liver Detoxification with Sulfite restricted diet for 2 weeks
- Nettle Root 300mg three times daily
- Testralin two daily
- Zinc 75 mg two daily
- Omega 10 three daily
- Vitamin D 5000IU Sublingual QD
- 8 oz. warm water with Sea Salt QAM
- No Alcohol
- No caffeine
- Restorative Sleep in bed by 10PM
- Nutrient Testing revealed deficiencies in zinc, calcium, and glutathione. Supplements added after testing are Zinc, Calcium and N-Acetylcysteine to assist body in making glutathione.
- Food Sensitivity Testing revealed sensitivities to casein, whey, cheese, milk, yogurt, asparagus, pears, chicken, and shrimp. These food items eliminated.
- Additional Genetic Testing for MTHFR genetic mutation reveals homozygosity for the A1298C MTHFR mutation 2 SNPs (single nucleotide polymorphisms)

Possible symptoms associated with A1298C MTHFR mutations:

- Hypertension
- Delayed speech
- Muscle pain
- Insomnia
- Irritable bowel syndrome
- Fibromyalgia
- Chronic fatigue syndrome
- Hand tremor
- Memory loss
- Headaches
- Brain fog

Possible signs associated with A1298C MTHFR Mutations:

- Elevated ammonia levels
- Decreased dopamine
- Decrease serotonin
- Decreased epinephrine and norepinephrine
- Decreased nitric oxide
- Elevated blood pressure
- Muscle tenderness
- Ulcers
- Pre-eclampsia

Possible conditions associated with A1298C MTHFR mutations:

- Fibromyalgia
- Chronic fatigue syndrome
- Autism
- Depression
- Insomnia
- ADD/ADHD
- Irritable bowel syndrome
- Inflammatory bowel syndrome
- Erectile dysfunction
- Migraine
- Raynaud's
- Cancer
- Alzheimer's
- Parkinson's
- Recurrent miscarriages

Subjective Patient Report

Feels drastic improvement inside 4-week period
No more brain fog or grey feelings, libido and sexual vigor have returned
Adapting well to new dietary lifestyle

Follow Up Lab at 90 days:

Liver panel: normal
CBC: normal
Lipid Panel: normal
Prolactin: 6.0
Cortisol AM: 17.0
LH: 4.6 mIU/mL
Total Testosterone: 802ng/dL
Free Testosterone: 18.0pg/mL

Sensitive Estradiol: 16.6pg/mL
DHT: 74ng/dL
SHBG: 32.0nmol/L
DHEA Sulfate: 379.0ug/dL
Vitamin D: 62.2ng/mL
TSH: 1.0 uIU/mL
fT3: 3.7 pg/mL
fT4: 1.09 ng/dL

Take Home Point

The eye only sees what the mind knows! Work with a physician experienced in optimizing male health and performance.

Chapter 9

Low Glycemic Nutrition – The Cornerstone of Health

All energy is neither created nor destroyed, it is merely transferred. This is the key phrase I want you to remember when it comes to nutrition and feeding your body. If you want to be lean, strong, and healthful then you have to feed your body energy. The energy I am talking about comes from eating food from the earth, not man made processed food. If you want great results with any exercise program, lifestyle change, or hormone optimization plan then you must obey the rule of energy transfer. Violate this rule and you will get mediocre results. Obey this rule, feed your body real food, establish and maintain healthy eating habits and YOU WILL ACHIEVE INCREDIBLE RESULTS.

The following **Low Glycemic/Nutrient Timed/Controlled Fasting** guideline will help you make the most of any testosterone restoration therapy program. Simply, replacing your hormones is not enough. If you are making lifestyle changes and/or attempting to naturally improve your hormone levels, this chapter will help as well.

Key Concepts in this Chapter:

- Low Glycemic Nutrition
- Nutrient Timing
- Controlled Fasting

This chapter is designed to enhance any natural program of hormone optimization, testosterone restoration therapy, exercise, and/or supplementation plan.

The purpose of this **Low Glycemic/Nutrient Timed/Controlled Fasting** chapter is to give you a guide that makes it easy to implement into your lifestyle. This chapter explains goals and gives the basic nutritional guidelines to help optimize your hormones.

Transitioning to Low Glycemic/Nutrient Timed/Controlled Fasting

Transitioning slowly helps you to adapt to a low glycemic, nutrient timed, controlled fasting lifestyle, which will give you control over your hormones. Nutrition is king when it comes to controlling not only your weight but also your health. Many people have food sensitivities they are not even aware of that affects their body in a negative way. This short transition will help you develop new habits and patterns, while allowing your body to reach its current peak abilities.

There can be an initial decrease in energy, which is sometimes experienced during the first week; this will subside as your body adapts to your powerful new low glycemic habits. After transitioning you may expand your food choices. It is a good idea to keep a food journal as well, noting your reactions to various foods. You will come to realize that there are foods, which provide you with incredible personal energy and others that do not. Stacking your nutrition with your "personal power foods" will give you that competitive edge.

Goals

Your Goal is Our Goal, Improve Strength, Energy, Libido and Fitness

- Improved Strength and Endurance
- Enhance your Libido
- Increase Metabolism and Energy
- Optimize your Hormones
- Be the best you can be

A specific goal of this **Low Glycemic-Nutrient Timed-Controlled Fasting** plan is to optimize human growth hormone levels. Growth hormone shares the same receptor site on cells as insulin. Having high insulin levels will decrease the uptake of growth hormone by the cells. Following a **LG/NT/CF** plan will keep your blood sugar low, which means stable insulin levels and higher levels of natural growth hormone.

The Two Pillars To Maintain Your Metabolism

The first is maintaining your lean muscle mass and you accomplish this by exercising daily with a combination of both strength training, also called resistance training, and aerobic exercise like running, cycling, swimming, dancing, hiking, and rowing. Exercise dramatically increases your energy expenditure, which helps you to rid yourself of excess body fat and increase important hormones, like epinephrine, which control lipolysis, which is the breakdown and utilization of fat for energy. Exercise also helps your body increase the number of mitochondria you have and improve the functioning of the mitochondria that already exist. These little powerhouses in each and every cell in the body are critical to your maintaining and improving your metabolism. The more you have and the more efficient they are the faster your metabolism and the easier it is to control your weight and increase your energy levels.

The second pillar is maintaining a balanced internal hormonal environment and this is accomplished by combining healthful daily nutritional habits with regular stressful exercise and supplementation with multivitamins and minerals. Maintaining a balanced internal hormonal environment starts with eating healthful, whole foods on a regular basis. These are the foods our bodies were designed to eat, foods that come from the earth, off a tree or bush and from animals. We were never designed to eat man made, highly processed foods loaded with additives and chemicals on a regular basis. Limiting or eliminating these from you diet will significantly improve your overall health and your metabolism.

So I am going to keep this short, simple and sweet since your nutrition plan has been created for you. The goal of this plan is to provide your body the energy it needs to perform the exercises in your workouts while also helping you to rid your body of excess, unwanted fat. You want to look and feel your best each and every day, so you have a very specific goal, which gives us a very specific nutrition plan. Perfect because the more specific the goal the easier it is to focus on our goal, which is to provide the right internal environment to power our bodies and get rid of the excess fat and optimize hormones.

Low Glycemic Nutrition

The cornerstone of all health is nutrition. Consuming foods that cause high blood sugar spikes will drop your testosterone production and the resultant high insulin levels from the high blood sugar will compete with growth hormone for the same receptor site. Other benefits of following low glycemic nutrition plans are: consistently high energy levels, eating satisfaction, efficient immunity, maintenance of healthy weight, and potential for increased longevity.

When a low glycemic meal is consumed, blood glucose elevates at a slower pace, allowing the pancreas to moderate the amount of insulin released so it is relative to the volume of glucose. Because there is less insulin circulating in the blood stream, fewer cells absorb glucose; levels never fall below optimal range. Food cravings and low energy crashes diminish once you adjust to the low glycemic diet, as the body is consistently able to utilize body fat as its primary source of energy. Consuming balanced, low glycemic meals maintains a consistent balance of hormone levels, allowing the body to function efficiently with optimal health.

Nutrient Timing or Carb Cycling

We are going to use a carb cycling plan that is timed with your daily workouts with a planned increase in calories at the end of the week. And it's money! Your lean proteins will come from sources like eggs, fish, chicken, turkey, beef and some dairy. Your carbohydrates are going to come from fruits, vegetables, oatmeal, and sweet potatoes. And your fats will come from nuts, olive oil and avocados. Oh.....and you'll have to eat a dozen sardines every day. Just kidding!
Your free meal, which comes once per week, this day is not an all-out feeding frenzy. But, feel free to have whatever you like for one meal, but do not stuff yourself. Remember to drink plenty of water and to take that 20-minute walk on your free day. Also, there is no alcohol on your free day. Remember, you want to power up your body not deplete it of energy!

So exactly how does this carb cycling work? Well research has demonstrated that alternating the amount of food every other day releases a protein called Sirtuin 1. And every organism tested demonstrated that calorie restriction lowered cancer rates, increased activity, decreased body fat weight, inflammation, disease and premature aging.

Sirtuin 1 also known as NAD-dependent deacetylase sirtuin-1 is a member of the sirtuin family of proteins. What is interesting about Sirtuin 1 and its activation is that it shows potential to increases fatty acid utilization, fat cell metabolism and mitochondriogenesis and decreases lipid profiles, lipiogenesis, adipogenesis, and inflammation in the intestines, lung and heart and also decreases neurodegeneration in the brain and central nervous system.

So exactly what does this mean? Well Sirtuin 1 acts to repair the damage done by the free radicals. It also helps the mitochondria to produce more energy and helps with weight loss by inhibiting fat storage and by increasing fat cell metabolism. All of these sounds like winners to me! All you have to do is eat more on the days we strength train and eat less on the days we train aerobically. And we do this by increasing and decreasing our natural starchy carbs on these days. It's really that simple!

Controlled Fasting or Intermittent Fasting

Fasting is defined as an act of willingly abstaining or reduction from certain or all food, drink, or both for a period of time. An absolute fast is normally defined as abstinence from all food or liquid for a defined period, usually a single day, or several days.

I know, "what do you mean don't eat"? Not quite, you get to eat, it's just that we like you to eat during a specific window of time during the day and then abstain from food during a period of time when you are most likely relaxing and preparing to rest for the evening. So, Why? Intermittent fasting boosts testosterone by increasing the expression of satiety hormones including insulin, leptin, adiponectin, glucagon-like peptide-1 (GLP-1), colecystokinin (CKK) and melanocortins, all of which are known to potentiate healthy testosterone actions, increase libido and prevent age-related testosterone decline. But what about eating breakfast? "Isn't it the most important meal of the day?" Well, breakfast just means to "break the fast" and we still are "breaking the fast" just a little later in the morning. It is still an important meal and I will get to that in just a minute.

So Let's Talk About Calories for a Minute

Calories or Food energy is the amount of energy obtained from food that is available through cellular respiration. Carbohydrates, proteins, and fats, all release energy during respiration—this is often called 'food energy'. When nutrients react with oxygen in the cells of living things energy is released. Calories are about energy. And when it comes to humans, energy that is not used is stored as fat.

So what does this mean for YOU and YOUR health: Eat too many calories and not enough exercise and calories get stored as fat. Eat the right amount of calories and exercise and your body takes energy from the stored fat when it needs more energy.

Think of calories as YOUR fuel when it comes to having energy to do the things YOU want to do. Think of the calories you put into your body as like the primary and reserve fuel tanks on a plane. When you eat your body uses the "fuel" you put into your stomach first, the primary tank, and then if it needs more "fuel" your body goes to your fat stores or reserve tanks for more "fuel". But it always uses what's in the primary tank first.

So a Calorie is a Calorie right?

Well this is where many people are confused and I at one time was no different! It turns out that this is not entirely true. Thanks to the field of nutrigenomics we now understand that all calories are not created equal and their effects on the human body can be quite dramatic and even have different effects on different people.

Studies have now revealed that diets that are made up of high glycemic carbohydrates that are rapidly absorbed sugars spike your blood sugar levels which in turn spike your insulin levels and constant high insulin levels promote fat gain, high triglycerides and cholesterol, insulin resistance, fatty liver, obesity, inflammation and all the disease associated with it.

So let's play a game I call *"Pick the Better Breakfast"*. Which one of these three breakfasts will supercharge your body giving it all the vitamins, minerals, and nutrients that it needs to power up your day, all while keeping your blood sugar levels stable. Here is the tricky part; they are all "healthful foods".

A. *Scrambled eggs with diced peppers on a bed of arugula with 10-grain bread sliced avocado and one cup of berries.*
B. *Steel cut oats with added flax, walnuts, and a cup of berries.*
C. *Rolled Oats with a cup of berries and a glass of orange juice.*

Picking the right one can make a huge difference as to whether you gain weight or lose weight. Seems pretty straight forward but there is actually an enormous difference in the way your body metabolizes the different foods you choose to eat each and every day.

You see foods that are digested quickly, enter the bloodstream quickly, which means higher blood sugars, which can mean a hormonal disturbance and weight gain. Compared to a food that is digested slowly which means more stable blood sugars, which means hormone balance. In addition some of these foods have anti-inflammatory properties and others inflammatory properties.

You see not all calories are not created equal. Let's take a look at a patient question. Tom asks: *Which is better for you apple juice or an apple?* Seems straight forward enough they are both made of the same food material right? Well, one enters the bloodstream very quickly because of its processing; the apple juice has had one of the important parts, the fiber, removed from it. However the apple in its natural state contains all of the vitamins, minerals, phytonutrients, antioxidants, and fiber! Everything your body needs. The rate at which the apple is digested is slower which means your body has time to utilize the energy from the apple. Eating apples promotes hormonal balance. Drinking juice can promote weight gain and hormonal imbalance.

In our examples of the 3 different breakfasts, they are all healthful foods. However that is where the similarity ends. You see each one of these breakfasts will be digested at different rates resulting in either rapid or slow escalation of blood sugar.

That difference alone can make all the difference in your overall health and in hormone balance. By maintaining stable blood sugars throughout the day you promote health, wellness, consistent energy, and utilization of digested and stored energy.

So which breakfast is our winner? While breakfast C is certainly healthy its consumption results in consuming roughly 80% more food later in the day than breakfast A. Breakfast B is certainly a healthy way to start the day, but its consumption led to eating 51% more food later in the day than breakfast A. Which makes breakfast A our winner!

The combination of eating eggs, peppers, arugula, avocado, and berries was not only a breakfast with low sugar content, but one with anti-inflammatory properties as well which means stable blood sugars, fats, insulin, and adrenaline levels. This group of foods sends a positive hormonal message.

The interesting fact here is that the types of food we eat not only supply our bodies with energy they also send distinctive hormonal messages. This is great news because we can directly control the foods we choose to eat.

Back to Controlled Fasting

I personally use a controlled fast daily as a way of giving my body a break from all the digestive work and as a way of giving myself freedom from food. It's amazing how much you can accomplish when you do not have to take breaks to eat.

You may think that you'll have no energy and that you will starve. But, quite the opposite happens. Your energy levels and productivity will soar! You will more than likely feel unbelievably energized too! You have more than enough energy stored in your body to exist for this very brief period, 12-18 hours without solid food. Heck, for 8 hours you will be sleeping anyways. During this controlled fast drink plenty of water with lemon to stay well hydrated. Also at any time during this period, you are in control, you can choose to end your controlled fast whenever you like and still have amazing benefits.

It's easiest to start with the simplest controlled fast, the 6pm to 6 am. You are asleep for most of this 12-hour period; you should be hitting the rack around 10 p.m. Then work your way to a 16-18 hour fast. You are always in control and can choose to end your fast whenever you like. When you choose to eat, remember to eat appropriately and not overeat. Chances are you will feel full quickly even with a small amount of food.

Planned Controlled Fasting Schedules:

Schedule 1: 6pm to 6am (beginners and the easiest)
Schedule 2: 6pm to 10 am (move from a 12 hour to 16-18 hour once every 2 weeks)
Schedule 3: 6pm to Noon
Schedule 4: 8pm to Noon
Schedule 5: Any 16-18 hour period that fits your schedule.

Short-term fasting has been shown to have the following health benefits, which were found after as little as 12-24 hours of fasting!

- Decreased body fat & body weight
- Maintenance of skeletal muscle mass
- Decreased blood glucose levels
- Decreased insulin levels & increased insulin sensitivity
- Increased lipolysis & fat oxidation
- Increased norepinephrine & epinephrine levels
- Increased glucagon levels
- Increased growth hormone levels
- Decreased food related stress
- Decreased chronic systemic Inflammation
- Increased cellular cleansing

These are all drinks that would be allowed during your fast:

- Black Coffee
- Green tea
- Herbal tea
- Water with lemon slice
- Sparkling Water

Low Glycemic-Nutrient Timed-Controlled Fasting Guidelines

1. EAT DURING A 8-10 HOUR PERIOD EACH DAY

- Eat 3 meals each day
- Have 2 snacks each day
- Eat lean proteins
- Keep to healthy fats
- Keep to low glycemic vegetables
- Eat the starch carbs in the hour after your workout

2. FAST FOR A 12-16 HOUR PERIOD EACH DAY

- 6 pm to 6 am is the easiest
- You may break your fast at any time, you are in complete control

3. DRINK PLENTY OF WATER

- Water, nonfrizzante or frizzante (only the Italians can make water sound so good!)
- Add a slice of lemon to your water
- Limit coffee to 1 cup in the morning
- Limit Green Tea to one cup daily
- Avoid soda and energy drinks
- Protein shakes as snacks

4. HAVE ONE "FREE MEAL" EACH WEEK

- Go for it!
- Do not over eat
- Have whatever your heart desires
- Some of you may require 2 free meals each week

What is Body Fat?

The body is made up of multiple components and not all weight is fat. There is water or fluid weight, excess materials, muscle, bone, and fat weight. Fat's main role is to provide a place for energy storage and it is highly efficient at doing so! One pound of fat roughly contains 3500 calories of stored energy, which is enough to walk almost 30 miles if your body could purely burn it. Ultimately to make a real impact we are talking about losing fat weight and keeping that super active metabolically demanding muscle. Men love to store fat viscerally and around the belly. They also can lose it very quickly. The most common type of fat storage we see in women is lower body fat storage, waist, hips, thighs, and buttocks. And a wonderful hormone known as estrogen, which is great from an evolutionary, reproductive standpoint gets accused of being the villain here. However, it's just not that simple because estrogen has both positive and negative effects depending on what tissue, what time of the month and what physiologic process we are discussing, and research shows that we are just beginning to understand fat cell metabolism and all of the numerous factors that control this complex hormonal process.

And as research progresses we are coming to realize that there is an incredible balancing act occurring between all the hormones in our bodies to control our weight. Hormones like thyroid, leptin, insulin, estrogen, testosterone, progesterone, atrial natriuretic peptide, glucagon, growth hormone, cortisol and the catecholamines: adrenaline and noradrenaline. Enzymes like, cyclical adenosine monophosphate, carnitine palmityl transferase and hormone sensitive lipase. Adrenorecptors in fat cells called apha-2 and beta-2 receptors and factors such as blood flow, transport, uptake and utilization.

Now, there is no such thing as targeted fat loss. However, a low glycemic diet combined with specific types of exercise is effective for liberating fat from these areas. You see low glycemic diets are great for inhibiting alpha-receptors in fat. Alpha-receptors are the "bad" receptors in fat and inhibiting them is good for fat loss. There is another kind of receptor in fat and these are called beta-receptors and they are the "good" receptors in fat. And you can activate them with the specific kinds of exercise you are going to perform and by using a little bit of caffeine. Warning!!! Taking more caffeine is not better and will not make you lose more weight or fat! You will just stress your adrenal glands and end up suffering from caffeinism. I'm not sure why I felt the need to include this very superficial, partial overview of a complex subject such as fat cell metabolism. I think it's just the fitness geek in me. Just know this....all YOU have to do is follow the plan.

Fat Cell Metabolism-The Unavoidable!

We all have fat cells and they are important for our bodies to function appropriately. Fat cells play a critical role in our immune system function. There are specific events that can occur in the life cycle of a fat cell. *Lipolysis* is the breakdown of fat in the fat cells to be used as energy. *Lipogenesis* is the formation of new fat in fat cells that occurs from eating way to many processed carbohydrates in particular and not getting enough exercise. And finally *hyperplasia*, which is an increase in the number of fat cells.

The life cycle of a fat cell is unavoidable and is why it is referred to as a futile cycle. The body is constantly breaking down fat for utilization and storing fat for future use. If you are eating more than what your body requires you will store the excess as fat and if you are eating less than what your body requires, your body will look to its fat stores for energy. It's really that simple.

Stopping Inflammation - another reason to eat Low Glycemic Foods

Guys love cars and cars have engines and so do our bodies. Your favorite car has an engine in it and that engine takes fuel to run it so you can go to the places you wanted to see. Well when the engine processes the fuel thru the act of combustion it gives of by-products collectively called emissions. Some of those emissions like water vapor are not so bad, but others like carbon monoxide are, and these emissions destroy the environment in which we live.

Well the trillion or so cells that make up our bodies each have an engine in them and theses engines are called mitochondria. Mitochondria take the nutrients from the foods that we eat and in turn, turn it into usable energy for the body. Well, in the process of generating this energy by-products are given off called free radicals. Some of these free radicals play an important role in cleaning up damaged cells in the body and others actually cause destructive processes to take place in the internal environment of our bodies.

Left unchecked these free radicals cause inflammation in the body and this is referred to as oxidative stress. Our bodies require an internal "catalytic converter", just like in a cars exhaust system, to clean up these dangerous, inflammatory causing free radicals, and they are called antioxidants. Antioxidants clean up the free radicals created by the mitochondria during the production of energy so the mitochondria can continue to produce energy efficiently and keep our bodies healthy. We get these antioxidants from the healthful foods that we eat on a regular basis and by supplementing our diet with vitamins and minerals.

If you have a very poor diet, then you will have a buildup of excess free radicals, and too many free radicals will lead to internal inflammation of the body. When the body becomes overrun with too much inflammation, chronic disease will set in inevitably.

Our bodies have other cleansing mechanisms, which are designed to clean up the waste products in the body, and the liver plays a major role in detoxification of free radicals. But when our bodies systems become overloaded with excessive levels of free radicals from oxidative stress, inflammation sets in and not far behind the inflammation is chronic disease.

Insulin Resistance

Insulin resistance is a condition where the cells in the body become resistant to the effects of insulin. This means higher levels of insulin are needed in order for insulin to have its effect. Now insulin is an amazing hormone with numerous roles but, chronic high levels of insulin in the bloodstream from poor dietary habits is bad. This can lead to different components of metabolic syndrome such as obesity, high blood pressure, high triglycerides, high glucose levels, inflammation, hormone derangement, and accelerated aging.

Insulin has multiple important roles in the regulation of our metabolisms one of which is the metabolism of fat. Insulin is primarily under the control of our diet and is easily affected by changing the quality and quantity of the carbohydrates we eat. Insulin levels will be reduced if you simply eat carbs that are lower on the glycemic index or reduce the quantity of the carbs that you eat. By addressing this issue from two different angles: reducing the quantity of starchy carbohydrate to every other day and limiting carbohydrates to vegetable only on the cardio days you can effectively control insulin and hence control its fat storage property when it is at higher levels in the bloodstream. Appropriate levels of insulin in the body have beneficial anabolic effects.

The major cause of insulin resistance is the lack of exercise and poor dietary habits, especially the consumption of excessive amounts of processed carbohydrates. Remember this, the poorer your dietary habits the more resistant you become to your insulin and your body has to make more insulin in an attempt to control your blood sugars and more insulin means more fat storage, hormone derangement, poorer health, and faster aging!

HIGH GLYCEMIC FOODS

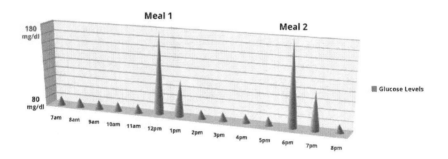

High glycemic processed foods like; cakes, cookies, candies, chips, bread, increase blood glucose quickly which results in high insulin levels. Because insulin is a "storage" hormone it promotes the absorption of sugar but insulin also inhibits cells from releasing their stores of fatty acids. Fatty acids comprise stored fat tissue. So when you have high insulin levels the body cannot use body fat as a source of energy.

What Happens When You Eat High Glycemic Foods?

- Unpredictable energy
- Food cravings
- Always hungry even though you just ate
- Unusual Fatigue
- Weight gain especially around the midsection

Now how about a diet that has low amounts of sugar and timed carbohydrates?

Low Glycemic Foods

On the other hand when a low glycemic food is eaten like apples, blueberries, celery, mushrooms, hummus, sweet potato, and quinoa, your blood glucose rises slower which allows the pancreas to release a smaller amounts of the storage hormone insulin. Since there is a smaller amount of insulin in the blood stream less glucose is absorbed. Because there are stabile insulin levels the body can utilize fat stores more efficiently.

Healthy Glucose Levels

Healthy frequent meals equal steady state glucose and insulin levels, increased metabolism and decreased cravings. Steady state glucose and insulin levels equal increased fat utilization and decreased fat production.

What Happens When You Eat Low Glycemic Fruits & Vegetables?

- High energy levels
- Strong immunity system
- Efficient metabolism
- Healthy Weight
- Optimized hormones
- Increased Growth Hormone

While You Are Transitioning

While you are transitioning to a healthier nutrition lifestyle you will eat minimal "starchy carbohydrates". (ie: sweet potatoes, squash, brown rice, black beans, quinoa) You will eat protein, healthy fats, and "fibrous carbohydrates", which have positive effects on blood sugar regulation. At the end of the book there is an appendix with tables of carbohydrates. The *carbs with the asterisks do not raise your blood sugars.* These are your "free carbs" that can be eaten at every meal.

Example: 6 scrambled eggs, (protein) 2 cups with a mix of onion, celery, mushroom, spinach, (free carbs) and 1 cup of avocado (healthy fat). The 2 cups of onion, celery, mushroom, and spinach are examples "free fibrous carbohydrate" that has numerous cardiovascular, endocrine, and digestive health benefits that promote healthy blood sugar metabolism. Eat these fibrous, healthy carbs freely.

How Many Calories Do You Need?

Here is a simple way of calculating your individual energy requirements. There are many formulas and adaptations of formulas. Whether you use this one or one on the Internet, pick one and calculate your specific dietary needs.

Everybody is different when it comes to the necessary number of calories they require to power their individual bodies. Just follow along here with this simple formula to know your specific nutritional needs. It's that simple. First you need to know your Ideal Body Weight and a very simple way to figure out your Ideal Body Weight is to use the HAMWI Formula for Ideal Body Weight.

Hamwi Formula For IBW (Ideal Body Weight):

Head over to http://www.americasfitnessdoctor.com/hamwi/ to see a video of Dr. Rob explaining the HAMWI formula.

If you are a man: 106 + 6 pounds for every inch over 60 inches.

If you are a woman: 100 + 5 pounds for every inch over 60 inches.

So if you are 5'8" man with a large frame: 106 + 6 x 8(48) = 154 pounds. If you have a large frame add 10 %, if you have a small frame subtract 10%. Our example has a large frame, so we calculate 154 x 10% = 15.4 + 154 = 169.4 pounds. Our example is 169.4 pounds, his IBW.

Now how many calories do you eat each day? The formula is very simple: On the days that you do strength training, multiply your IBW by 12. On the days that you do Interval Training, multiply your IBW by 10.

On the days our example does strength training, multiple IBW by 12. 169 x 12 = 2028 calories he need to consume for the day.

On the days our example is doing cardio for exercise, multiple IBW by 10. 169 x 10 = 1690 calories he needs to consume for the day.

Now there are 3 main food groups that you will build your nutrition from that are going to build that strong, healthy, fit body you want. Those groups of foods are called macronutrients. These consist of Proteins, Carbohydrates and Fats. But how much do you eat of each? I'm glad you asked because I have an answer for you:

30% Protein, 15% Carbohydrate and 55% Fat

OK, now our 5'8" male with an IBW of 169 consumes 2028 calories on the day he does strength training. So:

2028 calories x 30% protein = 608 calories from protein
2028 calories x 15% carbohydrates = 304 calories from carbohydrates
2028 calories x 55% fat = 1115 calories from fats

And 1690 calories on the day he does cardio exercises.

1690 calories x 30% protein = 507 calories from protein
1690 calories x 15% carbohydrates = 253 calories from carbohydrates
1690 calories x 55% fat = 930 calories from fats

Now convert your calories into grams as it will be much easier and you won't have to worry at all about counting calories. It's way easier to add up the grams from nutrition labels. And if you would like to know more one of my favorite sites to get nutrition information is nutritiondata.com.

9 calories per gram of Fat
4 calories per gram of Protein
4 calories per gram of Carbohydrate

Our 5'8" man with an IBW of 169 pounds who eats 2028 calories on Strength Training days needs:

Fat: 1115 calories /9 grams = 124 grams per day
Protein: 608 calories/ 4 grams =152 grams per day
Carbohydrates: 304 calories/4 grams = 76 grams per day

Our 5'8" man with an IBW of 169 pounds who eats 1690 calories on Cardio exercise days needs:

Fat: 930 calories /9 grams = 103 grams per day
Protein: 507 calories/ 4 grams =127 grams per day
Carbohydrates: 253 calories/4 grams = 63 grams per day
So how many times are we going to eat in in your 8-hour period? Most likely it will be 3 meals.

Now we divide our total grams we eat each day by 3. So our 5'8" man with an IBW of 169 pounds who eats 2028 calories on Strength Training exercise days needs:

Fat: 1115 calories /9 grams = 124 grams/3 = 41 grams per meal
Protein: 608 calories/ 4 grams =152 grams/3 = 51 grams per meal
Carbohydrates: 304 calories/4 grams = 76 grams/3 = 25 grams per meal

So our 5'8" man with an IBW of 169 pounds who eats 1690 calories on Cardio Exercise days needs:

Fat: 930 calories /9 grams = 103 grams/3 = 34 grams per meal
Protein: 507 calories/ 4 grams = 127 grams/3 = 42 grams per meal
Carbohydrates: 253 calories/4 grams = 63 grams/3 = 21 grams per meal

Calorie Worksheet

Step One: Calculate Your Ideal Body Weight (IBW)

106 + 6 x _____ inches over 60 inches = _____your Ideal Body Weight in pounds

If you have a large frame add 10%

If you have a small frame subtract 10%

Strength training multiply your IBW by 12. _____Your IBW x 12 =_____calories for the day

Interval Training multiply your IBW by 10. _____Your IBW x 10 =_____ calories for the day

Step Two: Calculate Your Calories

Strength Training Days

_____ Calories x 30% protein = _____calories from protein
_____ Calories x 15% carbohydrates = _____calories from carbs
_____ Calories x 55% fat = _____calories from fats

Interval Training /Cardio/Off Days

_____ Calories x 30% protein = _____calories from protein
_____ Calories x 15% carbohydrates = _____calories from carbs
_____ Calories x 55% fat = _____calories from fats

Step Three: Convert Your Calories Into Grams

Strength Training Days

Fat _____calories /9 grams = _____ grams per day
Protein _____calories/ 4 grams =_____grams per day
Carbohydrates _____calories/4 grams = _____grams per day

Interval Training /Cardio/Off Days

Fat _____calories /9 grams = _____ grams per day
Protein _____calories/ 4 grams =_____grams per day
Carbohydrates _____calories/4 grams = _____grams per day

Step Four: Calculate Your Grams Per Meal

Strength Training Days

Fat _____calories /9 grams = _____grams/3 = _____grams per meal
Protein _____calories/ 4 grams =_____grams/3 = _____grams per meal
Carbohydrates _____calories/4 grams = _____grams/3 =_____grams per meal

Interval Training /Cardio/Off Days

Fat _____calories /9 grams = _____grams/3 = _____grams per meal
Protein _____calories/ 4 grams =_____grams/3 = _____grams per meal
Carbohydrates _____calories/4 grams = _____grams/3 =_____grams per meal

Step Five: Starting The Transition

Strength Training Days:

Do not eat more than 100 grams of starchy carbohydrates out of you total carbs

Interval Training /Cardio/Off Days:

Do not eat more than 50 grams of starchy carbohydrates out of you total

Step Six: After Transition

Strength Training Days:

Do not eat more than 200 grams of starchy carbohydrates out of you total

Interval Training /Cardio/Off Days:

Do not eat more than 100 grams of starchy carbohydrates out of you total

Sample Meal Plan

<u>Training Day</u>

Breakfast: 6 scrambled eggs, (protein), 2 cups with a mix of onion, celery, mushroom, spinach, (free carbs) and 1 cup of avocado (healthy fat).

Lunch: 6 oz. of Beef Teriyaki (protein), 2 cups of Brussels sprouts and ½ cup of raw almonds (healthy fat).

EXERCISE: 2 scoop of whey protein before workout

Dinner: 5 oz. of grilled chicken breast, 12 asparagus spears light dressed with olive oil and sea salt, 1-cup sweet potato (starchy carb).

Evening Snack: 2 hardboiled eggs

Note Well: I eat all my starchy carbs after I exercise. This is known as "Back loading starchy carbs" to glycogen load my muscles. This keeps me stay low glycemic the entire day, optimizing hormone balance and ensuring I replenish muscle glycogen without increasing insulin dramatically.

Non-Training Day

Breakfast: 6 scrambled eggs, (protein), 2 cups with a mix of onion, celery, mushroom, spinach, (free carbs) and 1 cup of avocado (healthy fat).

Lunch: 6 oz. grilled tilapia (protein), 2 cups of lightly steamed Brussels sprouts, (free carbs) and ¼ cup of almonds

EXERCISE: Afternoon 20 minute walk

Dinner: 5 oz. grass fed beef (protein), 2 cups of lightly steamed broccoli/cauliflower mix (free carbs), 1-cup avocado (healthy fat) and ½ cup sweet potato (starchy carb).

Less Is More

Our ancestors ate nutrient-dense and calorie light foods such as fruits, vegetables, lean meats, and essential fats, with no refined or processed fats or simple carbohydrates. Human beings ate from what the earth provided. If it grew from the ground, fell from a tree, swam in a river, or ran through the woods, we killed it and we ate it.

Our DNA is of ancient design, unchanged over thousands of years, and modern food over the last 80 years has destroyed the health of generations. The rates of heart attacks, type II diabetes, obesity, strokes, hypertension, and gastrointestinal disorders in this country continue to explode. Adopting these healthful behaviors will drastically reduce the risks for all of these conditions.

Smart Tips

- Eat organic
- Eat free range and grass fed
- Avoid foods that are genetically modified
- Avoid artificial additives and preservatives.
- Consume foods from the earth not from a box
- Avoid foods stored in plastics
- Eat wild fish not farm raised
- Use Ezekiel bread over white bread
- Consume Natural peanut, almond, or cashew butter
- Limit portions to 6 ounces
- Eat your vegetables raw or steamed
- Choose low glycemic fruits like apples and berries
- Eat walnuts which are loaded with omega 3
- Consume avocado
- Eat olives
- Use extra virgin olive oil
- Use coconut oil
- Drink plenty of water
- Avoid artificial sweeteners
- Drink a full glass of water before you eat
- If you think you are hungry, drink water first you may just be thirsty
- Eat when you are hungry, stop when you are no longer hungry

Fuel for Your Body: Understanding the Macronutrients

First, I am going to discuss the macronutrients. These are the fuel for your body—eating the right portions of each macronutrient group will help you lose weight and maintain a healthy, active, lean body and optimize your hormones.

Proteins

The first macronutrient food group that I am going to talk about is proteins. I am not going to bore you with the things that happen to proteins when they are digested and how they fuel your body. Here are the important points. Proteins are the building blocks for tissue and proper immune function. Proteins are made up of amino acids. Some amino acids are called essential amino acids because the body requires them. Amino acids are the primary building blocks for new tissues in the body. Amino acids also enable vitamins to play a key role in the regulation of the body. Sources of complete proteins are eggs, turkey, beef, chicken, and fish. Eggs provide the optimal mixture of essential amino acids. Also, if one eats a variety of fruits, vegetables, and grains, all of the essential amino acids can be consumed.

Recommended Proteins:

Salmon	Swordfish	Duck	Lamb
Shrimp	Sardines	Pheasant	Egg Whites
Flounder	Tilapia	Greek Yogurt	Almond Butter
Sole	Grouper	Liver	Filet
Trout	Sea Bass	Turkey	Rabbit
Tuna	Bison	Chicken	Veal

Carbohydrates

The second macronutrient group is carbohydrates. Experts are always in disagreement as to how many carbohydrates should be consumed, but they are in agreement about one thing— carbohydrates are important fuel for your body if you are going to maintain an active healthy lifestyle. They help maintain protein in the body and help your central nervous system function properly. Not eating healthy carbohydrates will be detrimental to your goal of optimizing your hormones and will prevent your workouts from being productive.

Learning about carbohydrates can be confusing—there are just so many different kinds. They can be divided into simple versus complex, natural versus refined, starchy versus vegetable, slow versus fast and high glycemic index versus low glycemic index. But we are not going to worry about all these subcategories of carbohydrates. You do not need to understand all of that to make healthful choices.

First, let me discuss the carbohydrates that you must absolutely avoid to lose fat and optimize your hormones. These are man-made, refined carbohydrates. What are manmade, refined carbohydrates? Things like flour, chips, cakes, cookies, candies, crackers, bagels, pretzels, white bread, sugar, and syrup in all its forms (corn, maple, rice, brown, white, confectioners). After consuming refined carbohydrates, there is a large blood glucose surge. This leads to high levels of insulin, high levels of fat in the blood stream, and increased production of fat. Frequently eating refined carbohydrates decreases the body's response to insulin and the body's tissues become resistant to the positive effects of insulin. This results in the body requiring more and more insulin to control the consistently high blood sugar levels.

When the body can no longer make enough insulin to control the blood sugar, you get type 2 (insulin resistant) diabetes.

Conversely, fiber-rich carbohydrates, such as those in fruits, grains, and vegetables create lower blood glucose and insulin response and lower fat levels. These carbohydrates allow for the positive effects of insulin to occur, significantly decreasing the chances for weight gain.

Every meal should contain either a vegetable or fruit carbohydrate. When it comes to vegetable carbohydrates, the greener the better. For fruit carbohydrates, bear in mind that all fresh fruit is healthful, however keeping to the low sugar fruits like blueberries, raspberries, blackberries, strawberries, and apples will significantly improve your blood sugar levels.

Remember This: "You Can Not Out Train Poor Dietary Habits."

Look at the chart below for examples from each of the three healthful carbohydrate categories:

Vegetable Carbohydrates	Starchy Carbohydrates	Fruit Carbohydrates
Asparagus	Beans (navy, kidney, great & northern, black, pinto)	Apples
Artichokes	Breads (whole grain, Ezekiel, &wheat)	Banana
Broccoli	Potatoes (red, white)	All berries (blueberries, raspberries, strawberries)
Lettuce (herb mix, baby leaf, romaine, Italian mix)	Rice (brown), rice & quinoa &cereal, quinoa	All melons
Swiss chard	Yams or sweet potato	Dates
Mushrooms	Corn	Figs
Peppers (green, yellow, red)	Oatmeal (steel cut)	Grapes
Peas	Cream of wheat	Grapefruit
Tomatoes	Tortilla (gluten free)	Oranges
Spinach	Pastas (wheat & egg)	Pears
Zucchini	Red river hot cereal	Pineapple
Celery	Popcorn	Raisins
Cucumber	Squash (acorn, butternut)	Plums
Fennel	Hummus	Apricots
Cauliflower		

A-OK Fats for Life

Patients often ask me which fats are ok for their diet. I like to keep it simple and I have 3 fats that I really like and my body responds well to and they are easy to remember. **A-OK**, avocados, olive oil, and nuts. I know the "k" in nuts is silent. My 3 favorite nuts are almonds, walnuts, and pistachios. All of these fats are referred to as MUFAs or monounsaturated fats. These fats are found in a variety of plants, oils and nuts and are known to improve blood cholesterol and blood sugar levels, which improves circulation and can decrease your risk for heart disease and even cancers.

Avocados-are one I consider to be super foods that are versatile to use and taste great. Avocados contain a MUFA known as oleic acid, which is known to lower cholesterol, improve circulation, decrease heart attacks, decrease blood pressure, protect from strokes and are helpful in cancer protection. Avocados are full of vitamins, minerals, and antioxidants. My favorite way to have avocados is with scrambled eggs in the morning, but they are easy to add to any dish that you like and a great way to get your healthy fat for the day.

Olive Oil-This smooth flavorful monounsaturated oil contains a wide variety of antioxidants that are beneficial to your overall health. There is a large body of clinical evidence that 2 tablespoons of olive oil a day offers significant heart health benefits, decreased cholesterol, anti-clotting, anti-inflammatory and anti-hypertensive benefits. Something the Sicilians must already know! On my last trip to Sicily I saw a table of 90 year old plus men drinking olive oil and eating tangerines with black pepper. They must know something. I like to add olive oil to my protein drinks and use it as salad dressing. 2 tablespoons of extra virgin olive oil, half a fresh squeezed lemon, a clove of crushed garlic, and Italian spices and then whisk with a fork and Voila! Pour on top off some freshly stemmed vegetables, add to mashed cauliflower or use it on a salad.

"K" Nuts-Almonds, walnuts, and pistachios are at the top of my list of ways to get healthy fat. It is sufficiently and heavily documented that a diet, which includes these crunchy little powerhouses, makes it easier to lose weight and keep it off. Nuts are loaded with vitamins, minerals, and antioxidants. They are best consumed in their raw and natural state, so remember, no more than a handful at a time.

Healthy Fats:

- Almonds
- Pistachios
- Walnuts
- Olives (non-pitted)
- Olive oil, extra virgin
- Fish & Fish Oil
- Avocado
- Dr. Rob's salad dressing (2 tbsp. olive oil, crushed garlic, Italian seasoning, lemon and whisk)

There is another healthful fat referred to as PUFAs or polyunsaturated fats and these are also found in a variety of oils and plants. There is one in particular, called omega-3-fatty acids, an essential fatty acid, that is especially beneficial to your heart and is found in fatty fish like salmon, sardines, and walnuts. If you do not like eating these particular foods then supplementing with an omega-3-fatty acid is very beneficial.

Omega-3-fatty acids are also cardio protective by decreasing cholesterol, decreasing inflammation in blood vessels therefore decreasing plaque buildup, decrease blood clotting and decreasing overall body inflammation. Another important benefit to having a diet with plenty of omega-3-fatty acids is that it has been numerously documented that a diet rich in omega-3-fatty acids creates an environment idea for weight loss and hormone balance.

What's this glycemic index?

The glycemic index is a scale that measures the effects of food on blood sugar levels. Glucose is the base number of the index with a value of 100. Carbohydrates are given a numerical value relative to glucose on how fast they are broken down into glucose and moved into the bloodstream. The higher the number the faster it moves into the bloodstream and the lower the number the slower it moves into the bloodstream. A Dr. Jenkins from the University of Toronto developed this concept in the early 80's to help understand which foods were best for people with diabetes to eat. The body building community and health care professionals to manipulate fat loss has since used it widely. The hormonal concept is that when blood sugar is kept stabile then insulin levels are stable. Insulin is a storage hormone that when high encourages the storage of fat in the fat cells. Stabile insulin levels mean more energy and fewer cravings, which mean fat weight loss.

Foods with a high glycemic index, which is 70 and above are white bread, many breakfast cereals and white rice. Medium glycemic index carbohydrates, which are between 56-69, are sweet potatoes, basmati rice and whole-wheat products like pastas, bagels and more. Low glycemic foods are the majority of fruits and vegetables, oatmeal, brown rice, nuts, and legumes.

The majority of foods in the tables at the end of the chapter are low glycemic carbohydrates for this very reason. Maintaining stable insulin and blood glucose levels will lead to long-term success. There are times when I do utilize high glycemic carbohydrates like after a period of fasting prior to a workout to "frontload" carbs or after a particularly aggressive workout, like an endurance leg workout, when "back-loading" carbs is necessary to immediately shuttle nutrients into waiting muscle to promote growth and recovery.

Two Windows of Opportunity

There are two major windows of opportunity to feed your body. It is crucial to take full advantage of these times to care for your body. First is BREAKFAST and it literally means, "to break the fast". Your body has rested for the night and is primed and ready to be fed. But we are going to wait until 10am-12noon to eat to maintain our 16-18 hour fasting period. Feed it and feed it well. BREAKFAST IS THE FIRST IMPORTANT MEAL OF THE DAY; it's just that we wait to eat it!

The second most important meal of the day is in the hour immediately following your workout. Your body is primed again and ready to be fed within that golden hour after exercise. I like to use whey protein powder shakes right after exercise to feed my body. Whey protein is assimilated by the body at a faster rate, than casein protein powder.

Carbohydrates Are Best After Exercise (Back Loading Carbohydrates)

"Adrenaline, which is released during exercise from the adrenal glands and terminal nerve endings, remains active for approximately one hour post-exercise and suppresses insulin. This creates a one-hour time frame when starchy carbohydrates can be readily absorbed to replenish muscle glycogen without increasing insulin."

Now, just because you are eating healthy, doesn't mean it has to be boring. Spices are a great way to add flavor and help your body stay lean and trim. Here are **10** great ways to spice up your life and lose inches from your waist!

1. **Cinnamon**-the powerful antioxidants found in this sweet with heat spice help to keep blood sugar and your energy levels consistent. Add this to your morning oatmeal.

2. **Cayenne**-this fiery spice contains capsaicin, which helps to improve insulin sensitivity. Add this to your fish, chicken or vegetables.

3. **Coriander**-this lemony spice has a sedative effect that can help with insomnia and anxiety. Add this to any meat, chicken or fish.

4. **Ginger powder**-this tangy spice has anti-inflammatory properties that can aid sore muscles. Try adding this to vegetables sautéed in olive oil or ginger tea.

5. **Paprika**-this smoky hot spice has vitamin A in it, which aids in vision, immunity and bone growth. Try adding this to your eggs, chicken or fish.

6. **Chili Powder**-this fiery spice can help to decrease your appetite. Add this one to whatever you like!

7. **Curry Powder**-sweet tasting; has antioxidant properties that may help to reduce coronary artery disease. Add to fish, chicken, shrimp or beef.

8. **Saffron**-this red, slightly bitter spice may help to decrease PMS. Use this spice with chicken or lighter fish, like tilapia.

9. **Nutmeg**-this sweet spice contains myristicin that is known to help fight infections. Use this spice on top of butternut or acorn squash.

10. **Fennel**-this spice is one of my favorites! It has a licorice flavor. I prefer to use fresh fennel and slice it and grill it with olive oil. You can also make a fantastic sauce for pasta. Fennel aids in digestion and helps to freshen your breath. Here is my recipe; heat up 2 tablespoons of olive oil, add 2 cloves of chopped garlic and one finely chopped fennel bulb, add a little sea salt and black pepper. Top on a fine, long pasta and Voila!

The Importance of Supplementation

Everyone needs a good multivitamin and mineral supplement daily. The use of a multivitamin and mineral formula has the benefit of increasing your micronutrient profile by almost 40%. Vitamins are required by the body and are found in foods. Regardless of how healthful you try to eat supplementation with vitamins is required to obtain optimum health. Minerals are elements that come from the earth and must be ingested, as any living organism does not make them. An inadequate intake of the essential vitamins and minerals may increase the risk for cancer and other disease states.

The National Foundation for cancer research has stated that an inadequate intake of the essential vitamins and minerals may increase the risk for cancer. Their data has indicated that deficiencies in nutritional factors may contribute upwards of 60% of the cancer cases in the world today.

I highly recommend the daily use of vitamins and minerals. I encourage you to do your own research on this topic. I have found in my experience that the best formulations are found with small manufacturers of multivitamins and minerals.

*Nearly all of the supplements and Lifestyle Medicine Programs listed in this chapter are available at **http://www.alphamaleinstitute.com/the-alpha-male-store/***

* These statements have not been evaluated by the Food and Drug Administration. This product is not intended to diagnose, treat, cure, or prevent any disease.

Supplements

Citrus bioflavonoid complex

A large group of anti-oxidants found in citrus fruits that are sometimes referred to as Vitamin P. Citrus bioflavonoids are essential for the effective utilization of Vitamin C by the body. They are believed to have anti-inflammatory, anti-viral and anti-allergy properties.

Bilberry fruit extract

Bilberry fruit contains high concentrations of tannins, which are substances that act as an anti-inflammatory. This fruit also contains flavonoid compounds called anthocyanin, which have anti-oxidant properties. Anthocyanin helps to build strong capillaries and improve circulation throughout the body. The bilberry fruit has been associated with the care and treatment of atherosclerosis, cataracts, diabetes, diarrhea and vision disorders

Broccoli sprout extract

Broccoli sprouts contain a substance called sulforaphane. This substance is known to have anti-bacterial and anti-cancer properties. It can be found in cruciferous vegetables such as cauliflower, broccoli, cabbage, brussel sprouts and radish. Studies show that a diet rich in these cruciferous vegetables are beneficial to your health. Benefits of this extract include helping the body rid itself of toxins, alleviate allergy and asthma symptoms, boost the immune system, protect the skin from UV damage, and help reduce the risk of bladder, prostate and stomach cancer.

Chromium

Chromium is a team player with other elements to keep our metabolism running efficiently. It is estimated that the majority of Americans only get about half of what is needed. Chromium is needed to help maintain normal blood sugar.

Manganese

Manganese is a mineral element that plays an important role in numerous physiologic processes. Manganese plays a role in metabolism, bone development, wound healing and as the principal antioxidant in mitochondria. Insufficient levels of manganese have been associated with osteoporosis, glucose intolerance and epilepsy.

Vanadium

Vanadium is a trace mineral that is essential for maintaining a healthy body. Vanadium works in concert with molybdenum. Intriguing studies indicate that vanadium may help to normalize blood glucose levels, lower blood pressure, and enhance athletic performance. There are also studies that suggest that vanadium may help individuals with bipolar disorder.

Magnesium

Magnesium is involved in well over 300 metabolic reactions in the human body. Over 60% of the magnesium in the body is found in the skeleton and about 30% found in the muscle. Magnesium plays an important function in energy production, synthesis of molecules, cell signaling, iron transport, cell migration, and nutrient interactions. Deficiency in healthy individuals who are eating a healthy diet is rare as magnesium is abundant in both plant and animal sources. Magnesium can help to prevent hypertension, cardiovascular disease, osteoporosis, diabetes, migraines, asthma, and vascular disorders

Inositol

Inositol plays an important role in the body as it helps the nervous system to function. While it is not essential to the human diet, it helps to maintain cell membranes of highly specialized cells such as in the brain, eyes, bone marrow and intestines. Inositol helps to promote hair growth and may also have a role as an anticancer agent. People who drink caffeine or take numerous antibiotics may have an increased need for inositol because both these interfere with its effectiveness.

Selenium

Selenium is a trace element that is essential in small amounts. Selenium deficiency has been associated with an impaired immune system and increase progression of viral disease. There is a great deal of evidence that selenium reduces the incidence of cancer and that deficiency of selenium is associated with an increase in prostate and lung cancer.

Zinc

Zinc is an essential element for all forms of life. Zinc plays an important role in the structure of proteins and cell membranes. Numerous aspects of cellular metabolism are zinc dependent. Zinc plays a significant role in growth and development, neurologic function, immune response, testosterone production and reproduction.

Calcium

Calcium is the most common mineral in the human body. About 99% of calcium is found in the bones and teeth. Calcium is the major structural element in both bones and teeth. Calcium may help to prevent colorectal cancers, osteoporosis, hypertension, and premenstrual syndrome. Individuals with diets that have sufficient calcium intake are associated with a reduced incidence of being overweight.

Biotin

Biotin is a water-soluble vitamin that is required for enzymatic function in the human body. Deficiency is rare unless an individual is receiving parenteral feedings without biotin and in individuals who consume raw egg whites. Adequate biotin helps to prevent birth defects, diabetes, hair loss, and brittle fingernails.

Riboflavin

Riboflavin is a water-soluble B vitamin, also known as vitamin B2. Riboflavin also has oxidation-reduction (redox) functions, antioxidant functions, and nutrient interactions.

Vitamin B12

Vitamin B12 has the largest and most complex structure of all the vitamins. Methylcobalamin is required for the folate dependent enzyme, methionine synthase. This enzyme is required for the synthesis of the amino acid, methionine, from homocysteine. Inadequate function of this is associated with an increased risk of cardiovascular disease. Vitamin B12 deficiency affects 10-15% of people over the age of 60. Absorption of vitamin B12 from food sources requires normal function of the stomach, pancreas, and small intestine. Symptoms of vitamin B12 deficiency include megaloblastic anemia, neurologic symptoms, gastrointestinal symptoms, cardiovascular disease, dementia, Alzheimer's disease, increase incidence of breast cancer, and depression.

Vitamin B6

Vitamin B6 must be obtained from the food as humans cannot synthesize it. Vitamin B6 plays a vital role in over 100 enzymatic reactions. It is necessary for nervous system function, red blood cell formation and function, niacin formation, hormone function, and nucleic acid synthesis. Vitamin B6 helps to prevent cardiovascular disease, improve immune function, and cognitive function.

Niacin B3

Niacin is a water-soluble vitamin (also known as nicotinic acid or vitamin B3). Living organisms derive most of their energy from oxidation-reduction reactions (redox), which is a process involving the transfer of electrons. As many as 200 enzymes require the niacin coenzymes for redox-reactions. Niacin deficiency can result in pellagra, increased incidence of cancer, diabetes, cardiovascular disease, and high cholesterol.

Thiamin

Thiamin is a water-soluble B vitamin, aka (vitamin B1 or thiamine). Thiamin is necessary for enzymatic function. Deficiency of thiamin can lead to beriberi. Thiamin helps to prevent cataracts, Alzheimer's disease, congestive heart failure, and cancer.

Vitamin K

Vitamin K is a fat-soluble vitamin. Vitamin K is essential for the functioning of several proteins involved in blood clotting. Although vitamin K is a fat-soluble vitamin, the body store very little of it, and its stores are rapidly depleted without regular intake. Vitamin K is also important in bone mineralization, cell growth, osteoporosis, and cardiovascular disease.

Vitamin D

Vitamin D is a fat-soluble vitamin that is essential for maintaining normal calcium metabolism. Vitamin-D3 can be synthesized in humans by the skin by exposure to sunlight, or it can be obtained through diet. Vitamin D is also important for cell differentiation, immunity, insulin secretion, and blood pressure regulation. Deficiency of Vitamin D can lead to rickets, osteoporosis, osteomalacia, muscle weakness, colorectal cancer, breast cancer, depression, and pain.

Vitamin C

Vitamin C, also known as ascorbic acid, is a water-soluble vitamin. Humans do not make vitamin C, so we must consume it. Vitamin C is necessary for the synthesis of collagen. Collagen is an important structural component of blood vessels, ligaments, tendons, and bone. Vitamin C also plays an important role in the synthesis of norepinephrine, a neurotransmitter that is critical to brain function. Vitamin C is required for the synthesis of carnitine, which is essential for the transport of fat into cellular organelles called mitochondria, where fat is converted into energy. Vitamin C is a highly effective antioxidant. Vitamin C deficiency can cause scurvy. Vitamin C helps to prevent coronary heart disease, strokes, cancer, cataracts, gout, hypertension, diabetes, and helps to bolster the immune system.

Iodine

Iodine is a non-metallic trace element that is required by the human body for proper synthesis of thyroid hormones. Deficiency of iodine can lead to hypothyroidism, goiter, fatigue, weight gain, cold intolerance, and constipation.

Copper

Although copper is an essential trace element, supplementation is unnecessary as copper is found extensively in a wide variety of foods. The average dietary intake of copper on a daily basis exceeds the recommended dietary intake. There are studies that indicate that excess copper is associated with a decreased immune function, lower antioxidant status, increased atherosclerosis, and mental decline.

Folic acid

There is disturbing evidence that excess folic acid supplementation may encourage tumor growth. Folate is found naturally in grains, fruits, and vegetables, and in its natural state is of no concern and the preferred way of intake. There is sufficient folic acid added to numerous products that in combination with supplementation an individual can easily exceed the daily-recommended allowance.

Iron

While iron is an essential element, it is potentially toxic. Accidental iron overdose is the single largest cause of poisoning fatalities in children. Iron supplementation only needs to occur in a deficient state. Individuals at increased risk of iron deficiency are those with; chronic blood loss, pregnant, celiac disease, h. pylori infection, gastric bypass, strict vegetarians, and those who engage in regular intense exercise. It is recommended to have your iron levels checked to see if supplementation is necessary.

Beta Carotene and Vitamin A

Beta-carotene is the precursor to vitamin A. There is research to suggest that in excess it may increase the risk of cancer. The problem is believed to result when beta-carotene is ingested without other carotenoids that are present if it is ingested as real food. Once again, eat your fruits and vegetables. A person that is eating a reasonably healthy diet will be converting beta-carotene to vitamin A and as such supplementation is unnecessary. Vitamin A in excess is toxic to the liver and increases the risk of hip fracture.

Here is my list of the most important supplementation I believe every individual should be using on a regular basis to optimize their health. As we age and our nutritional habits and exercise choices change so does our additional supplementation requirement. But below is the basic daily supplementation I use daily regardless of my current exercise plan.

- Phyto-Multivitamin and Mineral Supplement
- Omega 3 Essential Fatty Acids purified and mercury free
- Ubiquinol/CoQ10
- Resveratrol
- Beverly International Quadracarn (a carnitine supplement)
- Vitamin D3 liquid 5000IU

I highly recommend discussing this supplementation list with your physician so you can tailor your supplementation needs to meet your nutritional requirements. Here is a list of additional herbal remedies and supplementation to utilize to optimize your health:

Ashwagandha

This Indian herb is a commonly used stress reducer and immune booster or adaptogen. The recommended dose is 150mg once or twice a day.

Capsaicin

This is an extract of cayenne pepper and can be used to reduce cholesterol and lower blood pressure, but is often used as a topical painkiller for arthritis. The supplement dose is measured in heat units.

Cinnamon

Recent studies have found cinnamon to be a potent aid in normalizing blood sugar in people with diabetes at doses of 1 to 2 grams. It can be taken as a supplement in capsule form.

Cocoa

My favorite of antioxidants! I like to use dark chocolate greater than 60% cocoa and limit to one ounce daily.

Bromelain

Bromelain is the most well-known anti-inflammatory enzyme. It is found in pineapple stems and helps in many inflammatory problems such as asthma, arthritis, and colitis. The dose is about 600 mg a day taken three times daily.

Fenugreek

Fenugreek can significantly lower blood sugar and blood fats. For people who have significant sugar problems, this can be a helpful herb.

Molybdenum

Molybdenum is a trace element that is found in several tissues of the body and is necessary for certain enzymatic activities to occur.

Ginger

This is another great addition to your day. I like to put it fresh ginger in my water. It can help thin the blood, lower cholesterol, and prevent nausea as well as act as a potent anti-inflammatory. Use fresh ginger in cooking or take ginger two to four 500mg capsules per day.

Ginseng

Panax ginseng-Chinese or Korean
Panax quinquefolius-American ginseng

There is some evidence that ginseng may help regulate insulin and blood sugar, and enhance immunity and adrenal function, as well as improve your ability to cope with stress. Take 200mg twice daily.

Green tea

This everyday beverage in china contains a class of compounds called polyphenols that boost liver detoxification and reduce cholesterol, inflammation, and oxidative stress, and can help prevent cancer and heart disease. Green tea is also thermogenic and may help increase metabolism and help with weight loss.

Quercitin

This potent plant bioflavonoid from onions and garlic and fruit has anti-inflammatory and antihistamine properties. In part it acts by preventing the release of histamine from mast cells and can help with food and environmental allergies.

Rhodiola

This relative newcomer to the herbal world of adaptogens is called Arctic root. It has few side effects and gently boosts energy and increases your resistance to stress.

Turmeric

This is the yellow spice commonly found in curry or yellow rice. It can be a powerful ally against inflammation and oxidative stress, useful in many inflammatory conditions.

Acetyl L-carnitine

This is another important amino acid that helps transport fat into the mitochondria for use. It has been shown to help prevent damage and improve the activity of mitochondria in aging. My favorite combination of carnitine is Beverly International's Quadracarn.

Alpha lipoic acid

Alpha lipoic acid is a powerful antioxidant and metabolic booster that has been shown to reduce blood sugar and prevent diabetic complications. It helps recycle the antioxidants, including vitamin C, E, and beta-carotene, making them more available to combat free radicals and help the body make more glutathione.

B Complex vitamins

Your need for B vitamins increases with every kind of stress. B vitamins help us improve the metabolism of stress hormones so we can process them. They are part of your basic multivitamin. However, some individuals require additional supplementation.

L-arginine

An essential amino acid that helps to dilate arteries, improves blood flow, and lowers blood pressure by increasing the body's natural production of nitric oxide. This increases the body's energy, strength, and endurance and may improve insulin resistance. Combined this with **Pycnogenol** which is French maritime pine bark which increases the body's natural production of nitric oxide and you have a potent combination that increases sexual function. *If you are using nitroglycerin this combination of supplements can induce low blood pressure. Please discuss with your Doctor before taking!*

Milk thistle

Milk thistle is sometimes used as a natural treatment for liver problems. These liver problems include cirrhosis, jaundice, hepatitis, and gallbladder disorders and to boost glutathione levels. Milk thistle may help to lower cholesterol and help with insulin resistance. Milk thistle may however mimic the effects of estrogen and if you are allergic to ragweed you may want to avoid its use.

Milk thistle is also known as silymarin. This is an old herbal remedy for liver disease that has been shown in controlled studies to improve liver function in people with alcoholic and infectious hepatitis. It works by increasing the synthesis of glutathione as an antioxidant and by increasing the rate of liver tissue regeneration. The standard dose is 70 to 210mg a day.

Coenzyme Q10

CoQ10 is a part of a critical step in the mitochondria involved in energy production, and helps boost metabolism. It also acts as an antioxidant. People who take the class of cholesterol-lowering drugs called statins deplete their CoQ10 levels because the same step in the body that produces cholesterol also produces CoQ10. In Parkinson's disease toxins damage the mitochondria. CoQ10 has been shown to slow or stop the progression of Parkinson's when given in high dosed (1200mg a day), without any side effects. It is my opinion that everyone over 40 should be taking CoQ10.

Creatine Powder or Chews

Creatine is another amino acid used for energy production in the mitochondria. It is commonly used by body builders to increase muscle mass. It can be used to build muscle and improve stamina and help your mitochondria produce energy. I personally use the chews, as they are not as gritty as the powder.

D-Ribose

This sugar is the raw material for energy production and the creation of ATP in the cells. It helps your mitochondria generate more energy along with carnitine and COQ10 and magnesium.

Vitamin C

We have no ability to increase our vitamin C production like most mammals can under stress. Taking extra vitamin C helps support your adrenal glands and your immune system during stress. There has also been good evidence that those with higher vitamin C levels excrete heavy metals such as lead and mercury easier. High doses of vitamin C can cause loose stools, if this occurs, stop the vitamin C.

GLA or gamma linolenic acid

This is one of the good and essential omega-6 fats that our body can't produce. It is helpful in reducing inflammation and can help lower blood pressure and cholesterol, as well as improve fat metabolism in people with diabetes. Taking one or two grams of GLA is a good way to get these essential fatty acids.

Glucomannan or konjac root fiber

This is the super fiber that is very viscous and soaks up fat, sugar, and water in the gut and reduces the overall glycemic load of any meal you eat. I have found this a powerful and safe way to promote weight loss, lower blood sugar and cholesterol.

Aspartic acid combined with magnesium

A dose of 400mg a day to help boost energy production in the mitochondria.

Magnesium

Magnesium is relaxation mineral. When we are stressed more magnesium is excreted in our urine. If we are deficient in magnesium we get headaches, constipation, palpitations, muscle cramps, and can become irritable. If you tend to be constipated, use magnesium citrate 150mg once to twice a day. If you have a sensitive stomach like me, use magnesium glycinate 150mg once a day.

N-acetylcysteine (NAC)

This amino acid-derived, sulphur-containing molecule is a key part of the way the body manufactures glutathione. Glutathione is produced by the liver and is the body's super hero recycling antioxidant. All toxins stick to glutathione to be removed from the body. In fact, it is used in emergency rooms to treat acetaminophen overdose and liver failure, and to prevent kidney failure for patients in hospitals getting X-rays or angiograms using dye, which can damage the kidneys. Taking this supplement can boost the body's own glutathione, which is one of the critical antioxidants that protect the mitochondria. N-acetyl cysteine can be used for detoxing heavy metals such as mercury and lead.

Probiotics

Use probiotic supplements, which include lactobacillus acidophilus, lactobacillus rhamnosis, and bifidobacteria. By restoring the normal gut flora they reduce overall immune activation and have been proven effective in many inflammatory diseases. They work by balancing the gut associated lymphoid tissue. Probiotics are found in the refrigerated section of most health food stores. Look for capsules containing 5 to 10 billion live organisms. Higher doses are often used in severe inflammatory conditions.

NADH

This is another little molecule the body makes that can get depleted, part of the critical energy production process in the mitochondria. This has been used effectively in patients with Chronic Fatigue Syndrome- a condition of malfunctioning and poisoned mitochondria. It can have an energy boosting and alertness effect like caffeine without the jitters. Take 5 to 20mg a day.

Zinc

Zinc is important for almost every function of the body, as well as in the normal function of the adrenal glands, modulating stress hormones and supporting the immune system. It is also one of the most common nutritional deficiencies. If you are feeling extra stressed take an additional 15 to 30mg of Zinc a day.

Dr. Rob's Fast Five Supplements for Leaning Out

CLA-Conjugated Linoleic acid helps to prevent the storage of fat you consume by forcing it to be burned for fuel. Take 2-3 grams with breakfast, lunch, and dinner.

Caffeine-Caffeine binds to the fats cells and encourages them to release more stored fat. There are multiple ways to get caffeine whether it is by pill or liquid. I recommend using it just before exercise to access its full benefit. No more than 300mg is necessary to accomplish this. Cycle your caffeine 21 days of use with 7 days

Decaffeinated Green Tea Extract-Green tea extract increases your metabolic rate, which allows your mitochondria to burn fat for fuel. Take 500mg 2-3 times per day.

Carnitine-helps to move fat to the mitochondria where the fat is burned away for good. Take 1-3 grams three times daily. My favorite combination of carnitine is Beverly International's Quadracarn.

Glucomannan-Amorphophallus konjac is a dietary source of fiber that will make you feel full and helps to bind fat, sugar, and water and eliminate them from your digestive tract. 1-3 capsules with water before a meal.

Dr. Rob's Fast Eight Supplements for Cellular Energy

D-Ribose - the raw material for the creation of ATP in the cells, which means creating energy. 1 scoop daily in 12 ounces of water or 1 chewable daily.

L-arginine - raw material that is needed by mitochondria for energy production.
1-2 pills daily.

Alpha-Lipoic Acid - 300 mg twice daily to help protect against free radicals.

D-Aspartic Acid - raw material that is needed by mitochondria for energy production. 1-4 750 mg capsules daily as recommended by manufacturer.

NAC(N-acetylcystiene) - an amino acid supplement that helps to restore the body's antioxidant levels. 600 mg capsule daily.

NADH - assists in the breakdown of fats and sugars and the production of ATP. 1 5-10 mg sublingual tablet daily.

Creatine Chews - is an amino acid used for energy production in the mitochondria. Tastes way better than the powder. 2-4 chewable tablets daily.

Essential Amino Acids - 3 tabs 3 times daily with meals. I prefer Beverly International's Density EAA Supplement

All of these are supplements that can fine tune your progress and take you to the next level but none of these supplements are as important as following the basic foundations of human health and wellness. *Eating healthy nutrition, regular meaningful exercise, drinking plenty of water, and getting appropriate periods of rest and sleep are the foundations of human health.*

I encourage you to talk with your Doctor about any and all of the supplements you wish to start taking.

All of the supplements listed in this chapter are available in our store **http://www.alphamaleinstitute.com/the-alpha-male-store/**

* These statements have not been evaluated by the Food and Drug Administration. This product is not intended to diagnose, treat, cure, or prevent any disease.

The Good and the Bad of Coffee/Caffeine

Ah, the almost indescribable aroma of freshly brewed espresso in the morning! I love the rush of chemicals in my brain as I inhale the chocolaty aroma and taste the fruity flavor of some earthy berry grown in a distant land. For me the act of making and drinking espresso in the quiet of the dark of the morning is such a calm way to start the day before the mad rush of ferrying children to school and dashing off to work.

You may also think coffee tastes good and it may get you going in the morning, but what will it do for your health?

There is a growing body of research shows that coffee drinkers, compared to nondrinkers, are less likely to have type 2 diabetes, Parkinson's disease, and dementia and have fewer cases of certain cancers, heart rhythm problems, and strokes. But, coffee is not proven to prevent these conditions.

It is possible that coffee drinkers have other advantages, such as better diets, exercise more, or have protective genes. So there isn't solid proof. But there are signs of potential health advantages and of course a few cautions.

If you're like the average American, who drinks an estimated 1.5 8-ounce cups of coffee each day you might want to know what all that caffeine is doing for you, or to you.

Coffee scores big points when it comes to the prevention of diabetes and the vast majority of studies on coffee have shown a distinct benefit when it comes to the prevention of diabetes. This holds true for both caffeinated, decaffeinated and tea drinkers.

It is believed that it is the very strong antioxidant capacity in coffee that provides the benefit. Also coffee contains minerals such as chromium and magnesium, which help the body regulate the hormone insulin. And we know consistent high levels of insulin are bad.

Studies reveal that coffee has been linked to lower risks for heart rhythm disturbances in men and women, and lower risk for strokes in women.

In a study of about 130,000 Kaiser Permanente health plan members, people who reported drinking 1-3 cups of coffee per day were 20% less likely to be hospitalized for abnormal heart rhythms than nondrinkers regardless of other risk factors.

A study of 83,700 nurses enrolled in the long-term Nurses' Health Study showed a 20% lower risk of stroke in those who reported drinking 2 or more cups of coffee daily compared to women who drank less coffee or none at all.

Coffee has also been linked to lower risk of Parkinson's disease, dementia, and Alzheimer's disease. A 2009 study from Finland and Sweden showed that, out of 1,400 people followed for about 20 years; those who reported drinking 3-5 cups of coffee daily were 65% less likely to develop dementia and Alzheimer's disease, compared with nondrinkers or occasional coffee drinkers.

Coffee consumption also has been linked to a decrease incidence of liver cirrhosis and liver cancer.

Coffee/Caffeine the Angelic Side

- Stimulate the release of dopamine, which helps us focus
- Increases lipolysis to use fat for energy
- Increases athletic performance
- Decreased incidence of diabetes
- Decreased incidence of neurocognitive disorders
- Decreased incidence of liver cancer
- Decreased incidence of stroke
- Decreased incidence of heart arrhythmias
- Decreased incidence of basal cell carcinoma
- Decreased incidence of depression
- Strong antioxidant capacity
- Boost sex drive

Coffee/Caffeine the Dark Side

Now what about the dark side of coffee/caffeine? A lot of patients ask me about coffee/caffeine. Caffeine is a drug like many others, and I recommend using it in a limited quantity. It is my opinion that one or two cups of coffee first thing in the morning is fine, but drinking caffeine throughout the day is something you want to avoid or you can end up with caffeinism.

Caffeinism, or caffeine intoxication, is a condition where you end up suffering with elevated blood pressure, rapid heartbeat, nervousness, insomnia, stomach cramps, muscle twitching, stomach upset, dehydration, stressed adrenal glands, and more. For those of you who are excessive caffeine drinkers, I would definitely wean yourself off of the caffeine. For example, if you are drinking six cups a day, I would decrease by one cup a day until you get to one or two cups daily.

Not everyone responds to caffeine the same way. Some people metabolize coffee differently than others and the gene involved is called CYP1A2. Our detoxification pathways are genetically determined. Which is why some people have one cup of coffee and are nervous and irritable and can't sleep for days and others like myself can have coffee any time of the day and sleep very well.

But this was not always the case. While I was in the Army in the 80's stationed in Germany I drank over "10 cups of Joe" every morning and I suffered from caffeine intoxication. So much so I could hardly hold a pen because my hands shook so much. I drank ridiculous amounts of coffee every morning mostly out of boredom. There's a lot of *"hurry up and wait"* in the military and I had a platoon sergeant that would reprimand us for reading books, but it was ok to smoke cigarettes and drink coffee while we sat and waited for our assignments for the day.

Coffee and Caffeine is most likely safe for most adults when used in **moderation**. However, caffeine can cause:

- Insomnia
- Nervousness and restlessness
- Anxiety
- Agitation
- Chest pain
- Headache
- Increased heart rate and respiration
- Stomach irritation (regular and decaffeinated coffees)
- Depletes neurotransmitters like dopamine
- Caffeine is a mild diuretic so it makes you urinate, which means you can become dehydrated faster

- Raises blood pressure
- Raises adrenaline
- Raises cortisol
- Raises homocysteine
- Nausea and vomiting

Caffeine can make these conditions worse!

- Anxiety
- Bipolar disorder
- Bleeding Disorders
- Heart conditions
- Diarrhea

- Irritable Bowel Syndrome
- Glaucoma
- High Blood Pressure
- Osteoporosis

A single cup of coffee with nothing added is about 15 calories. But start adding milk and sugar and the calories skyrocket to upwards of 500 in a single cup! So if you are trying to lose weight, remember this tip*: **Keep your coffee simple.***

Frappuccino w whipped cream	430 calories
Frappuccino	400 calories
Café late	165 calories
Café au lait	155 calories
Café mocha	570 calories
Cappuccino	150 calories
Carmel macchiato	320 calories
Coffee Black	15 calories

That being said there is evidence on *both sides of the fence* as to whether coffee/caffeine is good or bad for you. **What appears to be the key here is moderation**. So let me share my opinion with you, if you are a healthy adult, one or two cups of coffee a day is unlikely to hurt you. There is evidence to suggest that mild caffeine consumption aids in weight loss through increased lipolysis, which is the breakdown of fat in the fat cells, elevates your metabolism, may prevent cancer, diabetes and neurocognitive disorders because of antioxidant properties and increases athletic performance. Those all sound like winners to me, however if you are not a user of coffee or are sensitive to the effects of caffeine then it is best left on the shelf for someone else but you.

Alcohol - It's got to go to Boost Your Hormones

The great American institution that is the weekend party and there are endless reasons to party. Beloved by both men and women everywhere will destroy your hormone optimization goal period. My strong recommendation to you is to eliminate alcohol completely for the next 30 days. One night of tying one on with the jolly captain or favorite bandito will set you back 5-7 days.

This is what boozing it up will do to you during your transition period. It will slow the recovery of your body from the workouts you are doing daily. These workouts are depleting the glycogen stores in the liver and muscles, which mean your muscles are in need of repair post workout. Drinking alcohol absolutely stalls this recovery process. Alcohol causes your glycogen stores to go even lower and we need glycogen for repair and recovery.

Drinking alcohol means you are adding extra calories to your diet, not what you want to do. Now your body has to detox all the alcohol first before it gets around to burning off all the fats and carbs. Alcohol also increases the levels of the stress hormone cortisol, which promotes the storage of visceral or belly fat. Can you say, I'd like a muffin top or spare tire please? Alcohol also interrupts your sleep patterns and does not allow you to get adequate sleep because it decreases sleep duration and increases wakefulness during sleep. Because your sleep cycle is disrupted human growth hormone, which is partially responsible for muscle growth is reduced by up to 70%.

Alcohol's caustic properties also irritate the lining of the stomach, which in turns inhibits the absorption of nutrients. And because of alcohols diuretic effect, it makes you pee, you become dehydrated easily. Even minimal dehydration decreases your athletic performance and your ability to lose weight and boost your hormones. Alcohol during the next 30 days is best left on the shelf. This is a matter of priority and since you are reading this book your health must be a priority. So let's leave the booze alone for at least thirty days.

Here is a list of some alcoholic drinks and the amount of non-nutritional calories in just one drink:

Vodka—one shot	125 calories
Whiskey—one shot	125 calories
Tequila—one shot	115 calories
Southern Comfort—1.5 ounces	180 calories
Scotch—one shot	115 calories
Rum—one shot	125 calories
Bud Light	109 calories
Budweiser	146 calories
Coors	142 calories
Miller	152 calories
Miller Genuine Draft	148 calories
Amstel Light	93 calories
Wine, 4 ounces, white	90 calories
Cabernet	90 calories
Chardonnay	90 calories
Chianti	100 calories
Merlot	95 calories
Zinfandel	90 calories

Food Sensitivities

Despite following a healthful nutrition plan, many people have sensitivities to certain foods or food groups. These sensitivities can lead to reactions that cause symptoms such as headaches, runny nose, bloating, indigestion, cramps, constipation, diarrhea, belching, muscle aches and pains, brain fog and more.

An IgG Food Sensitivity Test will measure the presence of IgG antibodies to specific foods. If food specific binding occurs between the patient's IgG serum antibodies and the antigen protein then a symptomatic response to that food can occur causing symptoms and inflammation which can affect the persons overall health, wellness and hormones.

Eliminating these food sensitivities from you nutrition and rotating your food selections will decrease inflammation and help to improve nutrient assimilation in the digestive system leading to overall improved health and wellness - a necessary step in raising your hormones naturally.

On the following page is part of an IgG Food Sensitivity Test on a patient who was having constant bloating, gas, and severe abdominal distention after eating and difficulty losing weight. He had been to a gastroenterologist and had both an esophagogastroduodenoscopy (EGD), which is a test to examine the lining of the esophagus, stomach, and first part of the small intestine and a colonoscopy that both failed to disclose any disease process.

However on closer examination with food sensitivity testing we can see that he has significant dairy sensitivities to cheese, yogurt, milk, whey and casein proteins. Part of his daily routine was 2-3 protein shakes per day using casein protein powders. Upon elimination of casein protein shakes within 2 weeks his gastrointestinal symptoms had resolved and by the 6 week mark his weight decreased by 18 pounds. Simple elimination and rotation of foods can have profound impact on your overall health.

Comprehensive IgG Food Allergy Test + C. albicans, S. cerevisiae (94) - Dry Blood Spot

Dairy

Food	Value
Casein	6.29
Cheese	6.75
Goat Cheese	3.88
Milk	5.53
Mozzarella Cheese	6.57
Whey	5.05
Yogurt	4.82

Legumes'- Beans and Peas

Food	Value
Garbanzo Bean	2.80
Green Bean	2.63
Kidney Bean	3.54
Lentil	3.76
Lima Bean	2.38
Pea	2.66
Pinto Bean	3.33
Soybean	2.54

Fruit

Food	Value
Apple	2.78
Apricot	2.17
Banana	2.49
Blueberry	1.96
Coconut	3.18
Cranberry	2.17
Grape	2.35
Gliadin	2.87
Millet	2.84
Oat	2.41
Rice	1.79
Rye	1.97
Sorghum	2.05
Wheat Gluten	2.63
Wheat	2.08

Fish / Seafood

Food	Value
Cod Fish	3.03
Crab	2.29
Halibut	3.95
Lobster	2.18
Salmon	2.63
Sardine	1.87
Shrimp	1.81
Tuna	1.88

Meat/Fowl

Food	Value
Beef	2.81
Chicken	3.56
Egg White	3.57
Egg Yolk	2.88
Lamb	2.52
Pork	2.17
Turkey	2.39

Chapter 10

The Low T Book Get Lean & Strong Exercise Guide

The Low T Book Guide to Cardiovascular Days

This particular cardiovascular plan is highly effective for fast loss. Follow it as it is laid out. You are going to perform your aerobic plan 2 or 3 days each week. One of these days in the plan is an optional rest day; take it if you need it. Remember, more is NOT better. Let me repeat........MORE IS NOT BETTER. You will stress your body enough and more will just be overtraining and lead to one of two overtraining syndromes counterproductive to your hormone optimization goal.

The best time to perform your cardiovascular exercise is first thing in the morning in a fasted state. Why is this? There are numerous studies that document that cardiovascular exercise performed in a fasted state causes a massive increase in growth hormone. Human growth hormone is a herculean fat burner! It has also been documented that 30-second high intensity efforts increase human growth hormone by over 500% if performed properly. This means lean and strong men!

First, 30 minutes prior to exercise drink one 8 oz. cup of black coffee. If you do not tolerate caffeine or do not want to use it, it is ok and you will still get great results. Next, you will perform aerobic activity in 10-minute sections for a total of 30 minutes on 3 different pieces of aerobic equipment according to the following tables. You can choose from the following equipment: treadmill, stair-climber, elliptical, stationary cycle, rowing machine or jumping rope. I have found that the two best machines for this aerobic plan are the stair-climber and the treadmill. Every day that you do your cardiovascular exercise, change up the order of the equipment that you use. If Monday you went in the order of treadmill, stair-climber, rowing machine, on Wednesday change to rowing machine, treadmill and then stair-climber. Always mix up the order of the equipment on your 13 cardiovascular exercise days. If you only have access to one piece of equipment, such as a treadmill, that is fine to use for all 3 stages of exercise.

1st Machine for 10-minutes

10 minutes warm up at 50% effort

2nd Machine for 10 minutes

1:30 seconds @ 50% effort
30 seconds @ 90% effort
1:30 seconds @ 50% effort
30 seconds @ 90% effort
1:30 seconds @ 50% effort
30 seconds @ 90% effort
1:30 seconds @ 50% effort
30 seconds @ 90% effort
1:30 seconds @ 50% effort
30 seconds @ 90% effort

Rest For 3-5 Minutes And Drink 6-8 Ounces Of Cold Water

3rd Machine for 10-20 minutes

10-20 minutes at 50% effort

Ok, so what are 50% effort and 90% effort? Quite simply it is this:

50% effort: While running on the treadmill you have some difficulty holding a conversation with increased breathing. The effort is moderate.

90% effort: While running on the treadmill you CAN NOT hold a conversation. Slightly gasping for breath, the effort is hard.

Exercise Pausing and Increased Fat Loss

The type and intensity of exercise you perform directly affects how adrenaline and noradrenaline are released from the adrenal glands and the nerve terminals and this plays a major role in fat loss. Which is why I am such a fan of High Intensity Interval Training; it's short, it's fast, and it's done with great results.

But let's take a closer look as exercise intensity goes up so does the release of adrenaline and noradrenaline. Once you cross the lactate threshold then adrenaline and noradrenaline release explode. Now you'll notice that in the cardiovascular days I have you take a *5 minute break after your initial 20 minutes of HIIT* that's because there is a large release of fatty acids into the bloodstream about 5 minutes after your HIIT training ends.

Now if we do nothing those fatty acids that were released during the 5-minute break will be *re-stored* in the fat cell and in estrogen dominant men that means around the waist. So...that's why after your 5-minute break you get back on the treadmill and run at a slower pace about 50% effort for 10-20 minutes to utilize the free fatty acids floating in the bloodstream. Now they are gone for good and you are feeling lighter and leaner than ever! This simple strategy can literally bust you through any plateau in your training yet it is one of the least utilized.

The Low T Book Guide Strength Training Days

This particular strength-endurance training plan is highly effective for fast loss. Follow it as it is laid out. You are going to perform your strength-endurance training plan 4 days each week. More is NOT better. Let me repeat........MORE IS NOT BETTER. You will stress your body enough and more will just be overtraining and lead to one of two overtraining syndromes counterproductive to your weight loss goal.

The best time to perform your strength-endurance training days is in the afternoon around 4 to 6, so just after work for many of you. Why is this? The way I have your meals structured you will need the extra carbohydrates on your strength-endurance training days to achieve a highly effective workout. I have this staged accordingly for your complete success, just follow the plan.

There are 3 strength phases to moving a weight: The lifting phase, lowering phase and the holding phase. The holding phase is the strongest, the lower phase is the next strongest, and the lifting phase is the least strong. You can change the pace of the reps for all the phases to stimulate your muscles and cause muscle adaptation. The rate of the repetition can be anywhere from 4-6 seconds.

Your one rep pace should be a 6 second count with a slight pause at the end of the lifting phase. *So perform a 3 count during lifting phase, pause, and then a 3 count in lowering phase.* Choose a weight that is 40-65% of your one rep max weight with proper form. You should be able to complete between 13 and 18 repetitions. If you cannot complete 13 repetitions then the weight is too heavy and if you complete 18 reps without any fatigue the weight is too lite. The total time under tension for each set will be greater than 70 seconds. This type of strength endurance training will stimulate type 1a muscle fibers, which will help to create a strong, lean athletic physique. Lean and mean. Evolutionarily speaking it's not the biggest and strongest that survives, it's the most efficient.

This 30-day plan rotates carbohydrate volume daily. On strength training days you will be eating approximately 100 grams of carbohydrates, on aerobic training days you will be eating approximately 50 grams of carbohydrate. After 2 weeks you may increase your carbohydrates to 200 grams on strength training days and 100 grams on aerobic training days. At any time you can use this rotational plan to control your weight, always keeping yourself within striking distance of your best body.

The Warm Up

Prior to each Strength-Endurance Training session perform this warm up. Use a weight that is 30% of your max weight. Take a 30 second rest between exercises.

PUSH UP-20 REPS
BODYWEIGHT SQUATS-20 REPS
2 POINT DUMBBELL ROW-20 REPS
KNEE UPS-50 REPS
CURL AND PRESS-20REPS

The Low T Book Guide Exercises

Body-Weight Squat
Stand tall with your feet shoulder-width apart, arms straight in front of you at shoulder level. Keep your chest up and engage your core by pulling your belly towards your spine and lower your body by bending your knees and pushing your hips back, stop. Then slowly push yourself back up to the starting position.

Burlesque Squat
With or without weight stand with your heels on a 2 inch piece of wood with your feet together engage your core by pulling your belly towards your spine. Squat down until your thighs are parallel with the floor then slowly raise yourself back up again.

Single Leg Calf Raises
Standing on the edge of a step or the cross bar of an incline bench with the balls of your feet planted firmly on the step and your heel hanging over the edge engage your core by pulling your belly towards your spine and raise your heel a few inches above the edge of the step so you are on your tiptoe. Hold the position for a moment and then lower your heel below the edge of the step and repeat. To add weight to this exercise hold a dumbbell on the same side as the calf you are exercising.

Dumbbell Lunge with Bicep Curl
While holding dumbbells at your side step your right foot forward and bend your knee until your thigh is parallel to the floor and as you lunge curl the weights up the reverse and return to start and repeat with the left leg.

Dumbbell Step Ups
Stand in front of a bench with your feet shoulder width apart, bend at your knee then step onto the bench. Step down to the floor and then repeat.

Reverse Dumbbell Lunge
While holding dumbbells at your side step your left foot backwards and bend your knee until your thigh is parallel to the floor. Remember to engage your core by pulling your belly towards your spine. Return to the start position and repeat on the other side.

Forward Dumbbell Lunge
While holding dumbbells at your side step your left foot forward and bend your knee until your thigh is parallel to the floor. Remember to engage your core by pulling your belly towards your spine. Return to the start position and repeat on the other side.

Single Leg Lunge
Place one leg behind you on the bench and extend the other leg out in front. With your hands on your hips lower yourself to the floor making sure your extended leg becomes parallel to the floor then push yourself back up. After you finish the number of reps, switch to the other side.

Reverse Lunge and Sweep
Stand with your feet shoulder width apart and your hands clenched in fists in front of your face. Lunge back with your left leg in a slight curtsy fashion then rise back up shifting your weight to your right leg and then sweep your left leg out and up to touch your right hand, put your left arm behind you for balance. Repeat till reps are finished and then switch to the other leg.

Dumbbell deadlift
Start by picking up the dumbbells at your feet and pulling the weights up with the backs of your legs until you are standing up straight then return back to the starting position but stopping about 6 inches from the floor before you return back up.

Abdominal Wheel Rollout
This classic piece of equipment will help you strengthen your abdominals. Master this beginning exercise rolling out from your knees; make sure there is padding under your knees, keep your chin tucked, your arms straight and pull your stomach into your spine as you rollout keeping your core tight. As you improve you can start from your feet.

Alternating Knee Lift
Lift the right knee up to your waist level touching your knee to your right hand. Return to the start position and repeat on the left side. Focus on keeping your core tight and pulled into your spine. You can add intensity by increasing the speed but remember to stay in control.

Two Point Dumbbell Row

Holding a dumbbell in one hand assume a two point stance with your feet shoulder width apart and stagger the foot on the weight side slightly behind the opposite foot. Rest your nonworking hand on either knee or unsupported in the air. Maintain the natural arch to your spine and pull the dumbbell straight up your side keeping the dumbbell close to your body and then lower. If you feel too much pressure in your low back decrease the amount of weight.

Dumbbell Upright Row

Stand with your feet shoulder width apart. Engage your core by pulling your belly towards your spine. Palms of your hands facing you pull the dumbbells straight up using your elbows and stop when your elbows are slightly above the level of your shoulders. Return to the start position.

Dumbbell Face Pulls

Holding dumbbells in both hands stand with feet shoulder width apart and bend at the waist until your chest is parallel with the floor. Engage your core by pulling your belly towards your spine. Let your arms hang straight down from your shoulders with palms facing you and lift dumbbells towards the sides of your forehead simultaneously squeezing your shoulder blades together and then lower the dumbbells. You can also perform this exercise lying chest down on an incline bench to remove the pressure off your lower back.

Dumbbell Lawn Mower Pull

Holding a dumbbell in your right hand palm facing you assume a two point split stance with your feet shoulder width apart and stagger the foot on the weight side behind the opposite foot. Engage your core by pulling your belly towards your spine. Bend your left knee and hips until they are about 45 degrees to the floor and let the dumbbell hang out in front. Then rotate your torso and row the dumbbell to your shoulder return to start and repeat on the opposite side.

Standing Dumbbell Shoulder Press

Stand with your feet shoulder width apart. Engage your core by pulling your belly towards your spine. Lift the dumbbells to your shoulders (start position) then with palms facing outwards press the weight overhead. Return to the start position and repeat.

Seated Dumbbell Shoulder Press

Sit with your feet flat on the floor. Engage your core by pulling your belly towards your spine. Lift the dumbbells to your shoulders (start position) then with palms facing outwards press the weight overhead. Return to the start position and repeat.

Incline Triceps Extension

Set your bench to a 30-45 degree angle. Sit back on the bench with both feet flat on the floor. Engage your core by pulling your belly towards your spine. Keeping your elbows in tight and your upper arm perpendicular to the floor lower the dumbbell towards the sides of your forehead then contract your triceps to extend your elbows overhead. Repeat on other side.

Two Point Triceps Kickbacks

Holding a dumbbell in one hand assume a two point stance with your feet shoulder width apart and stagger the foot on the weight side slightly behind the opposite foot. Rest your nonworking hand on either knee. Engage your core by pulling your belly towards your spine. Keeping your elbows in tight and your upper arm parallel to the floor and palm facing you raise the dumbbell by straightening your arm until it is parallel with the floor.

Standing Dumbbell One Arm Triceps Extension

Stand with your feet shoulder width apart. Engage your core by pulling your belly towards your spine. Hold the dumbbell in your right hand and lift overhead keeping upper arm and elbow close to your head and lower dumbbell in an arc behind your head then raise dumbbell back up to the starting position. Repeat on opposite side.

Biceps Curl and Press

Standing begin by keeping your chest up engage your core by pulling your belly towards your spine with a bilateral biceps curl then bring the weights to your shoulders rotating the palms of your hands outward and then push the weights overhead. Returning to the start position is one repetition.

Hammer Curl

Stand with feet shoulder width apart. Engage your core by pulling your belly towards your spine. Turn your hands so your palms face each other and lift the weights to your shoulders focusing on keeping your elbows stationary. Do not "swing" the weights.

Incline Biceps Curl

Set your bench to a 30-45 degree angle. Sit back on the bench with your arms hanging straight down and your hands facing forward. Curl the dumbbells upwards towards your shoulders while keeping your upper arms still. Pause at the top position and slowly lower.

Dumbbell Concentration Curl

Either sitting or standing raise the dumbbell with the biceps muscle to the front of the shoulder just before the apex of the movement rotate your wrist outward ending the lifting phase with concentration on the long head of the biceps muscle. Return to the start position and lift with the opposite arm.

Pushup

Start your pushup in the up position with your feet together and your hands slightly wider than your shoulders. Engage your core by pulling your belly towards your spine. Your body should be straight from your head to your feet. Lower your body till your chest almost touches the floor, pause and then push yourself back up to the starting position.

Heart to Heart Pushup

Start the pushup in the up position with your feet shoulder width apart and your hands together beneath your chest. Engage your core by pulling your belly towards your spine. Your body should be straight from your head to your feet. Lower your body till your chest almost touches the floor, pause and then push yourself back up to the starting position.

Wide-Hands Pushup

Start the pushup in the up position with your feet together and your hands twice shoulder width apart. Engage your core by pulling your belly towards your spine. Your body should be straight from your head to your feet. Lower your body till your chest almost touches the floor, pause and then push yourself back up to the starting position.

Close-Hands Pushup

Start the pushup in the up position with your feet together and your hands closer than shoulder width apart. Engage your core by pulling your belly towards your spine. Your body should be straight from your head to your feet. Lower your body till your chest almost touches the floor, pause and then push yourself back up to the starting position.

Plank

Start in a pushup position then bend your elbows and rest your weight on your forearms, your body will form a straight line then squeeze your core as if you were about to be punched in the stomach and hold for 30 seconds. Do this eight to ten times.

Kettle bell or Barbell Swing

Stand with your feet a little more than shoulder width apart, squat down and grab the kettle bell or dumbbell, thrust your hips forward, straighten your knees and swing the weight up to the level of your chest then let the weight return back down between your legs and swing back up.

Incline Dumbbell Fly

Set your bench to a 30-45 degree angle. Sit back on the bench with both feet flat on the floor. Engage your core by pulling your belly towards your spine. Hold dumbbells with palms facing one another. Extend your arms above your chest with arms slightly bent. Lower your arms out to your sides about shoulder level and contract your chest muscles to bring your arms together.

Dumbbell Squat and Press

Start with your feet shoulder width apart, hold the weights at your shoulders with your elbows bent, bend at your knees and squat to the floor, then as you stand back up press the weights over your head until your arms are straight and return to the start position.

Dumbbell Chest Press

This can be performed with a bench or a stability ball. With your feet flat on the floor, hold the weights by your chest with your elbows bent and palms facing forward. Press the dumbbells towards the ceiling then return back to start.

Incline Dumbbell Chest Press
Performed with an incline bench. Place your feet flat on the floor and hold the weights by your chest with your elbows bent and palms facing forward. Press the dumbbells towards the ceiling then return back to start.

Alternating Dumbbell Chest Press
This can be performed with a bench or a stability ball. With your feet flat on the floor, hold the weights by your chest with your elbows bent and palms facing forward. Alternate pressing the dumbbells towards the ceiling then return back to start.

Standing Alternating Front Dumbbell Raise
Holding a pair of dumbbells, stand with your feet shoulder width apart and dumbbells at your side. Engage your core by pulling your belly towards your spine. Using either palms facing you or palms down grip lift the dumbbell on your right side raising your arm straight out in front of you until parallel with the floor pause and return. Repeat on the other side.

Lateral Dumbbell Raises
Holding the weights by your side with palms facing you engage your core by pulling your belly towards your spine and lift the weights to the level of your shoulders and then slowly lower.

Dumbbell Front Raises
Holding the dumbbell in front of you with palms facing inwards engage your core by pulling your belly towards your spine and lift the dumbbell to the level of your shoulders and then slowly lower.

Bent Dumbbell Lateral Raises
Bending at the waist hold the weights under your shoulders with palms facing you engage your core by pulling your belly towards your spine and lift the weights to the level of your shoulders and then slowly lower.

T-Stabilization
Start in the pushup position, keeping your arms straight and your core engaged shift your weight onto your right arm and rotate your torso and reach your left arm into the sky so that your body forms a T. Pause then return to start and repeat on the other side.

Ski Jump

Start in the semi squat position with your feet shoulder width apart and your arms in front of you like you are holding ski poles. As you stand up raise onto your toes and bend your arms at the elbows kicking your arms back then return to start.

Push Up Rows

Get into the push up position with your hands gripping the dumbbells and your feet about shoulder width apart. You can perform a pushup or not then pull one dumbbell to the side of your chest lower it then repeat on the other side.

Squat and Thrust or Burpee

With your feet shoulder width apart then bend your knees to put your hands on the floor and then thrust your legs back into a pushup position. Quickly return to the standing start position.

Hip Raise

Lie on the floor on your back with your knees bent and your feet flat on the floor then squeeze your glutes and raise your hips into the sky until your body forms a straight line pause and then lower to the starting position.

Plank Alternating Knee to Elbow

Start in the pushup position with your hands under your shoulders engage your core by pulling your belly towards your spine and bring your right knee to your left elbow and pause and then return and bring your left knee to your right elbow and pause repeat 8-10 times.

Mountain climber

Start in the pushup position and engage your core by pulling your belly towards your spine and then quickly alternating your knees to your chest as if you are running.

Single Leg Romanian Deadlift

Stand with your feet shoulder width apart then raise your right foot off the floor and extend your right arm in front of you. Bend forward at the hips and keep your back flat and raise your right leg behind you so your body forms a T. Then return to the start position and repeat for the given number of reps then do the other side.

30-Day Countdown to the Low T Book Lean and Mean Body

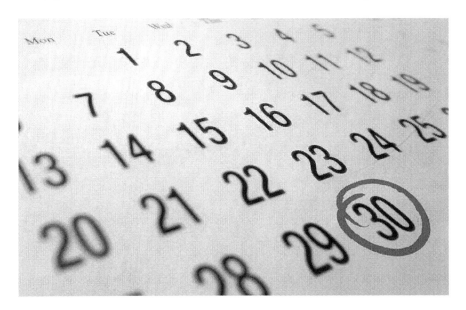

Note: All strength training day meals and snacks are interchangeable with other strength training day meals and snacks. Likewise, all aerobic training day meals and snacks are interchangeable with other aerobic training day meals and snacks.

Day 30- The Low T Book Strength Training Day Meals

Meal 1
Two large organic eggs with ½ cup of egg whites scrambled and one diced pepper, 1 tsp of crushed red pepper on a bed of 2 cups of spinach or arugula 2 slices of multigrain toast with butter (22 grams of carbs)
1 cup of halved strawberries (12 grams of carbs)

Snack
1 medium apple (20 grams of carbs) and 2 scoops of protein pudding

Meal 2
4-6 ounces of a lean protein (chicken breast, turkey, tuna, salmon, beef) on a bed of 2 cups of mixed leaf lettuces or spinach or romaine lettuce (2 grams of carbs) with a teaspoon of extra virgin olive oil and fresh lemon squeezed or 1 tbsp. of apple cider vinegar
1 medium apple (20 grams of carbs) or half a sweet potato

Snack
15 raw almonds or walnuts (4 grams of carbs)

Meal 3
4-6 ounces of a lean protein (chicken breast, turkey, tuna, salmon, beef)
2 cups of broccoli lightly stemmed (24 grams of carbs) or 2 bunch of broccoli rabe or 2 cups of brussel sprouts.

Snack
¼ cup of cottage cheese with ¼ of blueberries (7 grams of carbs) or 2 scoops of protein pudding

Water
_____12ounces	_____12ounces
_____12ounces	_____12ounces
_____12ounces	_____12ounces
_____12ounces	_____12ounces

The Low T Book Strength Training Exercise

Dumbbell Concentration Curls

Set 1_____, Set 2 _____

Pushup

Set 1_____, Set 2 _____

Incline Dumbbell Curls

Set 1_____, Set 2 _____

Dumbbell Upright Row

Set 1_____, Set 2 _____

Standing Dumbbell Shoulder Press

Set 1_____, Set 2 _____

Incline Dumbbell Fly

Set 1_____, Set 2 _____

Plank

30 secs_____, 30 secs_____, 30 secs_____, 30 secs_____, 30 secs_____, 30 secs_____

Perform 2 sets of these exercises.

Set 1: 13-18 reps,

Set 2: 13-18 reps. <30 seconds rest between sets and 60 seconds rest between exercises.

Choose a weight that is 40-65% of your one rep max weight with proper form.

When performing the Plank you will hold the position for 30 seconds then rest for 10 seconds and repeat 4-6 times.

Fat Burning Finishing Exercise:

Kettle bell/barbell swing-perform 4 sets of 25 reps

Set 1_____, Set 2 _____, Set 3_____, Set 4____

Day 29- The Low T Book Aerobic Day Meals

Meal 1
Protein shake
½ cup of organic lactose free milk (7 grams of carbs)
1 scoop of protein powder (4 grams of carbs)
½ cup of blueberries or ½ cup of strawberries (10 grams of carbs)
¼ teaspoon of cinnamon
Add 1 cup of water, 3-5 ice cubes and blend in mixer

Snack
5.3-ounce container of plain Greek yogurt with ¼ cup of added fruit (10 grams of carbs) or 2 scoops of protein pudding

Meal 2
4-6 ounces of a lean protein (chicken breast, turkey, tuna, salmon, beef) on a bed of 2 cups of mixed leaf lettuces or spinach or romaine lettuce (2 grams of carbs) with a teaspoon of extra virgin olive oil and fresh lemon squeezed or 1 tbsp. of apple cider vinegar

Snack
15 raw almonds or walnuts (4 grams of carbs)

Meal 3
4-6 ounces of a lean protein (chicken breast, turkey, tuna, salmon, beef) 2 cups of cauliflower lightly stemmed and mashed with ½ teaspoon of olive oil (12 grams of carbs) or 12 asparagus spears.

Snack
¼ cup of cottage cheese with ¼ of strawberries (3 grams of carbs) or 2 scoops of protein pudding

Water
_____12ounces		_____12ounces	
_____12ounces		_____12ounces	
_____12ounces		_____12ounces	
_____12ounces		_____12ounces	

The Low T Book Guide Cardiovascular Exercise

1st Machine for 10-minutes

10 minutes warm up at 50% effort

2nd Machine for 10 minutes

1:30 seconds @ 50% effort
30 seconds @ 90% effort
1:30 seconds @ 50% effort
30 seconds @ 90% effort
1:30 seconds @ 50% effort
30 seconds @ 90% effort
1:30 seconds @ 50% effort
30 seconds @ 90% effort
1:30 seconds @ 50% effort
30 seconds @ 90% effort

REST FOR 3-5 MINUTES AND DRINK 6-8 0UNZES OF COLD WATER

3rd Machine for 10-20 minutes

10-20 minutes at 50% effort

Day 28- The Low T Book Strength Training Day Meals

Meal 1
2 large eggs with ½ cup of egg whites scrambled with 1 teaspoon of crushed red pepper ¼ cup steel cut oats & ¼ red river cereal. After you cook it add cinnamon and/or nutmeg & 5 almonds (20 grams of carbs)
1 cup of halved strawberries (12 grams of carbs)

Snack
1 medium apple (20 grams of carbs) and 2 scoops of protein pudding

Meal 2
4-6 ounces of a lean protein (chicken breast, turkey, tuna, salmon, beef) on a bed of 2 cups of mixed leaf lettuces or spinach or romaine lettuce (2 grams of carbs) with a teaspoon of extra virgin olive oil and fresh lemon squeezed or 1 tbsp. of apple cider vinegar
1 medium apple (20 grams of carbs) or half a sweet potato

Snack
15 raw almonds or walnuts (4 grams of carbs)

Meal 3
4-6 ounces of a lean protein (chicken breast, turkey, tuna, salmon, beef)
2 cups of broccoli lightly stemmed (24 grams of carbs) or 2 bunch of broccoli rabe or 2 cups of brussel sprouts.

Snack
¼ cup of cottage cheese with ¼ of blueberries (7 grams of carbs) or 2 scoops of protein pudding

Water
_____12ounces   _____12ounces
_____12ounces   _____12ounces
_____12ounces   _____12ounces
_____12ounces   _____12ounces

The Low T Book Strength Training Exercise

Bench Step Ups	**Perform 2 sets of these exercises.**
Set 1_____, Set 2 _____	Set 1: 13-18 reps
Deep Knee Burlesque Squats	Set 2: 13-18 reps. <30 seconds rest between sets and 60 seconds rest between exercises.
Set 1_____, Set 2 _____	
Dumbbell Deadlift	Choose a weight that is 40-65% of your one rep max weight with proper form.
Set 1_____, Set 2 _____	

Reverse Dumbbell Lunge

Set 1_____, Set 2 _____

Squat and Press

Set 1_____, Set 2 _____

Incline Dumbbell Press

Set 1_____, Set 2 _____

Abdominal Wheel Rollouts

Set 1_____, Set 2 _____

Fat Burning Finishing Exercise:

Kettle bell/barbell swing-perform 4 sets of 25 reps

Set 1_____, Set 2 _____, Set 3_____, Set 4_____

Day 27- The Low T Book Aerobic Day Meals

Meal 1
Oatmeal Protein Pancakes:
2 scoops of protein powder mixed with ¾ cup of egg whites, ¼ teaspoon of cinnamon, one tablespoon of oats (10 grams). Add enough water for batter type consistency, spray skillet with cooking spray. Top with sugar free syrup or butter. (10 grams of carbs). 1/2 cup of strawberries (6 grams of carbs)

Snack
5.3-ounce container of plain Greek yogurt with ¼ cup of added fruit (10 grams of carbs) or 2 scoops of protein pudding

Meal 2
4-6 ounces of a lean protein (chicken breast, turkey, tuna, salmon, or beef) on bed of 2 cups mixed leaf lettuces or spinach or romaine lettuce (2 grams of carbs) with a teaspoon of extra virgin olive oil and fresh lemon squeezed

Snack
15 raw almonds or walnuts (4 grams of carbs)

Meal 3
4-6 ounces of a lean protein (chicken breast, turkey, tuna, salmon, beef) 2 cups of cauliflower lightly stemmed and mashed with ½ teaspoon of olive oil (12 grams of carbs) or 12 asparagus spears.

Snack
¼ cup of cottage cheese with ¼ of strawberries (3 grams of carbs) or 2 scoops of protein pudding

Water
_____12ounces   _____12ounces
_____12ounces   _____12ounces
_____12ounces   _____12ounces
_____12ounces   _____12ounces

The Low T Book Guide Cardiovascular Exercise

1st Machine for 10-minutes

10 minutes warm up at 50% effort

2nd Machine for 10 minutes

1:30 seconds @ 50% effort
30 seconds @ 90% effort
1:30 seconds @ 50% effort
30 seconds @ 90% effort
1:30 seconds @ 50% effort
30 seconds @ 90% effort
1:30 seconds @ 50% effort
30 seconds @ 90% effort
1:30 seconds @ 50% effort
30 seconds @ 90% effort

REST FOR 3-5 MINUTES AND DRINK 6-8 0UNZES OF COLD WATER

3rd Machine for 10-20 minutes

10-20 minutes at 50% effort

Day 26- The Low T Book Strength Training Day Meals

Meal 1
Two large organic eggs with ½ cup of egg whites scrambled and one diced pepper, 1 tsp of crushed red pepper on a bed of 2 cups of spinach or arugula 2 slices of multigrain toast with butter (22 grams of carbs)
1 cup of halved strawberries (12 grams of carbs)

Snack
1 medium apple (20 grams of carbs) and 2 scoops of protein pudding

Meal 2
4-6 ounces of a lean protein (chicken breast, turkey, tuna, salmon, beef) on a bed of 2 cups of mixed leaf lettuces or spinach or romaine lettuce (2 grams of carbs) with a teaspoon of extra virgin olive oil and fresh lemon squeezed or 1 tbsp. of apple cider vinegar
1 medium apple (20 grams of carbs) or half a sweet potato

Snack
15 raw almonds or walnuts (4 grams of carbs)

Meal 3
4-6 ounces of a lean protein (chicken breast, turkey, tuna, salmon, beef)
2 cups of broccoli lightly stemmed (24 grams of carbs) or 2 bunch of broccoli rabe or 2 cups of brussel sprouts.

Snack
¼ cup of cottage cheese with ¼ of blueberries (7 grams of carbs) or 2 scoops of protein pudding

Water
_____12ounces		_____12ounces	
_____12ounces		_____12ounces	
_____12ounces		_____12ounces	
_____12ounces		_____12ounces	

The Low T Book Strength Training Exercise

Close Hand Push ups

Set 1_____, Set 2 _____

Standing Dumbbell One Arm Triceps Extensions

Set 1_____, Set 2 _____

Seated Dumbbell Press

Set 1_____, Set 2 _____

Dumbbell Upright Row

Set 1_____, Set 2 _____

Dumbbell Triceps Kickbacks

Set 1_____, Set 2 _____

Standing Dumbbell Front Raise

Set 1_____, Set 2 _____

Plank

30 secs_____, 30 secs_____, 30 secs_____, 30 secs_____, 30 secs_____, 30 secs_____

Perform 2 sets of these exercises.

Set 1:13-18 reps

Set 2:13-18 reps. <30 seconds rest between sets and 60 seconds rest between exercises.

Choose a weight that is 40-65% of your one rep max weight with proper form.

Fat Burning Finishing Exercise:

Kettle bell/barbell swing-perform 4 sets of 25 reps

Set 1_____, Set 2 _____, Set 3_____, Set 4_____

Day 25- The Low T Book Aerobic Day Meals /Optional Exercise OFF Day

Meal 1
Protein shake
½ cup of organic lactose free milk (7 grams of carbs)
1 scoop of protein powder (4 grams of carbs)
½ cup of blueberries or ½ cup of strawberries (10 grams of carbs)
¼ teaspoon of cinnamon
1 cup of water, 3-5 ice cubes and blend in mixer

Snack
5.3-ounce container of plain Greek yogurt with ¼ cup of added fruit (10 grams of carbs) or 2 scoops of protein pudding

Meal 2
4-6 ounces of a lean protein (chicken breast, turkey, tuna, salmon, beef) on a bed of 2 cups of mixed leaf lettuces or spinach or romaine lettuce (2 grams of carbs) with a teaspoon of extra virgin olive oil and fresh lemon squeezed or 1 tbsp. of apple cider vinegar

Snack
15 raw almonds or walnuts (4 grams of carbs)

Meal 3
4-6 ounces of a lean protein (chicken breast, turkey, tuna, salmon, beef) 2 cups of cauliflower lightly stemmed and mashed with ½ teaspoon of olive oil (12 grams of carbs) or 12 asparagus spears.

Snack
¼ cup of cottage cheese with ¼ of strawberries (3 grams of carbs) or 2 scoops of protein pudding

Water
_____12ounces   _____12ounces
_____12ounces   _____12ounces
_____12ounces   _____12ounces
_____12ounces   _____12ounces

The Low T Book Guide Cardiovascular Exercise

1st Machine for 10-minutes

10 minutes warm up at 50% effort

2nd Machine for 10 minutes

1:30 seconds @ 50% effort
30 seconds @ 90% effort
1:30 seconds @ 50% effort
30 seconds @ 90% effort
1:30 seconds @ 50% effort
30 seconds @ 90% effort
1:30 seconds @ 50% effort
30 seconds @ 90% effort
1:30 seconds @ 50% effort
30 seconds @ 90% effort

REST FOR 3-5 MINUTES AND DRINK 6-8 0UNZES OF COLD WATER

3rd Machine for 10-20 minutes

10-20 minutes at 50% effort

Day 24- The Low T Book Strength Training Day Meals

Meal 1
2 large eggs with ½ cup of egg whites scrambled with 1 teaspoon of crushed red pepper
¼ cup steel cut oats & ¼ cup red river cereal. After you cook it add cinnamon and/or nutmeg & 5 almonds (20 grams of carbs)
1 cup of halved strawberries (12 grams of carbs)

Snack
1 medium apple (20 grams of carbs) and 2 scoops of protein pudding

Meal 2
4-6 ounces of a lean protein (chicken breast, turkey, tuna, salmon, beef) on a bed of 2 cups of mixed leaf lettuces or spinach or romaine lettuce (2 grams of carbs) with a teaspoon of extra virgin olive oil and fresh lemon squeezed or 1 tbsp. of apple cider vinegar
1 medium apple (20 grams of carbs) or half a sweet potato

Snack
15 raw almonds or walnuts (4 grams of carbs)

Meal 3
4-6 ounces of a lean protein (chicken breast, turkey, tuna, salmon, beef)
2 cups of broccoli lightly stemmed (24 grams of carbs) or 2 bunch of broccoli rabe or 2 cups of brussel sprouts.

Snack
¼ cup of cottage cheese with ¼ of blueberries (7 grams of carbs) or 2 scoops of protein pudding

Water
_____12ounces	_____12ounces
_____12ounces	_____12ounces
_____12ounces	_____12ounces
_____12ounces	_____12ounces

The Low T Book Strength Training Exercise

Standing Calf Raises

Set 1_____, Set 2 _____

Dumbbell One Leg Calf Raises

Set 1_____, Set 2 _____

Dumbbell Lawn Mower Pulls

Set 1_____, Set 2 _____

Bicep Curl and Press

Set 1_____, Set 2 _____

Standing Dumbbell Lateral Raises

Set 1_____, Set 2 _____

Dumbbell Face Pulls

Set 1_____, Set 2 _____

Abdominal Wheel Rollouts

Set 1_____, Set 2 _____

Perform 2 sets of these exercises.

Set 1: 13-18 reps,

Set 2: 13-18 reps. <30 seconds rest between sets and 60 seconds rest between exercises.

Choose a weight that is 40-65% of your one rep max weight with proper form.

Fat Burning Finishing Exercise

Kettle bell/barbell swing-perform 4 sets of 25 reps

Set 1_____, Set 2 _____, Set 3_____, Set 4_____

Day 23- The Low T Book Aerobic Day Meals

Meal 1
Oatmeal Protein Pancakes
2 scoops of protein powder mixed with ¾ cup of egg whites, ¼ teaspoon
of cinnamon, one tablespoon of oats (10 grams). Add enough water for
batter type consistency, spray skillet with cooking spray. Top with sugar
free syrup or butter. (10 grams of carbs). 1/2 cup of strawberries (6 grams
of carbs)

Snack
5.3-ounce container of plain Greek yogurt with ¼ cup of added fruit (10
grams of carbs) or 2 scoops of protein pudding

Meal 2
4-6 ounces of a lean protein (chicken breast, turkey, tuna, salmon, beef)
on a bed of 2 cups of mixed leaf lettuces or spinach or romaine lettuce (2
grams of carbs) with a teaspoon of extra virgin olive oil and fresh lemon
squeezed or 1 tbsp. of apple cider vinegar
Snack
15 raw almonds or walnuts (4 grams of carbs)

Meal 3
4-6 ounces of a lean protein (chicken breast, turkey, tuna, salmon, beef)
2 cups of cauliflower lightly stemmed and mashed with ½ teaspoon of
olive oil (12 grams of carbs) or 12 asparagus spears.

Snack
¼ cup of cottage cheese with ¼ of strawberries (3 grams of carbs) or 2
scoops of protein pudding

Water

_____12ounces		_____12ounces	
_____12ounces		_____12ounces	
_____12ounces		_____12ounces	
_____12ounces		_____12ounces	

The Low T Book Guide Cardiovascular Exercise

1st Machine for 10-minutes

10 minutes warm up at 50% effort

2nd Machine for 10 minutes

1:30 seconds @ 50% effort
30 seconds @ 90% effort
1:30 seconds @ 50% effort
30 seconds @ 90% effort
1:30 seconds @ 50% effort
30 seconds @ 90% effort
1:30 seconds @ 50% effort
30 seconds @ 90% effort
1:30 seconds @ 50% effort
30 seconds @ 90% effort

REST FOR 3-5 MINUTES AND DRINK 6-8 0UNZES OF COLD WATER

3rd Machine for 10-20 minutes

10-20 minutes at 50% effort

Day 22- The Low T Book Strength Training Day Meals

Meal 1
Two large organic eggs with ½ cup of egg whites scrambled and one diced pepper, 1 tsp of crushed red pepper on a bed of 2 cups of spinach or arugula 2 slices of multigrain toast with butter (22 grams of carbs) 1 cup of halved strawberries (12 grams of carbs)

Snack
1 medium apple (20 grams of carbs) and 2 scoops of protein pudding

Meal 2
4-6 ounces of a lean protein (chicken breast, turkey, tuna, salmon, beef) on a bed of 2 cups of mixed leaf lettuces or spinach or romaine lettuce (2 grams of carbs) with a teaspoon of extra virgin olive oil and fresh lemon squeezed or 1 tbsp. of apple cider vinegar
1 medium apple (20 grams of carbs) or half a sweet potato

Snack
15 raw almonds or walnuts (4 grams of carbs)

Meal 3
4-6 ounces of a lean protein (chicken breast, turkey, tuna, salmon, beef) 2 cups of broccoli lightly stemmed (24 grams of carbs) or 2 bunch of broccoli rabe or 2 cups of brussel sprouts.

Snack
¼ cup of cottage cheese with ¼ of blueberries (7 grams of carbs) or 2 scoops of protein pudding

Water
_____12ounces		_____12ounces	
_____12ounces		_____12ounces	
_____12ounces		_____12ounces	
_____12ounces		_____12ounces	

The Low T Book Strength Training Exercise

Front Dumbbell Raises

Set 1_____, Set 2 _____

2 point Dumbbell Row

Set 1_____, Set 2 _____

Wide Hand Push ups

Set 1_____, Set 2 _____

Standing Shoulder Press

Set 1_____, Set 2 _____

Dumbbell Triceps Kickback

Set 1_____, Set 2 _____

Plank

30 secs_____, 30 secs_____, 30 secs_____, 30 secs_____, 30 secs_____, 30 secs_____

Perform 2 sets of these exercises.

Set 1:13-18 reps,

Set 2:13-18 reps. <30 seconds rest between sets and 60 seconds rest between exercises.

Choose a weight that is 40-65% of your one rep max weight with proper form.

Fat Burning Finishing Exercise:

Ski Jump-perform 4 sets of 25 reps

Set 1_____, Set 2 _____, Set 3_____, Set 4_____

Day 21-The Low T Book Aerobic Day Meals /Optional Exercise OFF Day

Meal 1
Protein shake
½ cup of organic lactose free milk (7 grams of carbs)
1 scoop of protein powder (4 grams of carbs)
½ cup of blueberries or ½ cup of strawberries (10 grams of carbs)
¼ teaspoon of cinnamon
Add 1 cup of water, 3-5 ice cubes and blend in mixer

Snack
5.3-ounce container of plain Greek yogurt with ¼ cup of added fruit (10 grams of carbs) or 2 scoops of protein pudding

Meal 2
4-6 ounces of a lean protein (chicken breast, turkey, tuna, salmon, beef) on a bed of 2 cups of mixed leaf lettuces or spinach or romaine lettuce (2 grams of carbs) with a teaspoon of extra virgin olive oil and fresh lemon squeezed or 1 tbsp. of apple cider vinegar

Snack
15 raw almonds or walnuts (4 grams of carbs)

Meal 3
4-6 ounces of a lean protein (chicken breast, turkey, tuna, salmon, beef) 2 cups of cauliflower lightly stemmed and mashed with ½ teaspoon of olive oil (12 grams of carbs) or 12 asparagus spears.

Snack
¼ cup of cottage cheese with ¼ of strawberries (3 grams of carbs) or 2 scoops of protein pudding

Water
_____12ounces   _____12ounces
_____12ounces   _____12ounces
_____12ounces   _____12ounces
_____12ounces   _____12ounces

The Low T Book Guide Cardiovascular Exercise

1st Machine for 10-minutes

10 minutes warm up at 50% effort

2nd Machine for 10 minutes

1:30 seconds @ 50% effort
30 seconds @ 90% effort
1:30 seconds @ 50% effort
30 seconds @ 90% effort
1:30 seconds @ 50% effort
30 seconds @ 90% effort
1:30 seconds @ 50% effort
30 seconds @ 90% effort
1:30 seconds @ 50% effort
30 seconds @ 90% effort

REST FOR 3-5 MINUTES AND DRINK 6-8 0UNZES OF COLD WATER

3rd Machine for 10-20 minutes

10-20 minutes at 50% effort

Day 20- The Low T Book Strength Training Day Meals

Meal 1
Two large organic eggs with ½ cup of egg whites scrambled and one diced pepper, 1 tsp of crushed red pepper on a bed of 2 cups of spinach or arugula 2 slices of multigrain toast with butter (22 grams of carbs) 1 cup of halved strawberries (12 grams of carbs)

Snack
1 medium apple (20 grams of carbs) and 2 scoops of protein pudding

Meal 2
4-6 ounces of a lean protein (chicken breast, turkey, tuna, salmon, beef) on a bed of 2 cups of mixed leaf lettuces or spinach or romaine lettuce (2 grams of carbs) with a teaspoon of extra virgin olive oil and fresh lemon squeezed or 1 tbsp. of apple cider vinegar
1 medium apple (20 grams of carbs) or half a sweet potato

Snack
15 raw almonds or walnuts (4 grams of carbs)

Meal 3
4-6 ounces of a lean protein (chicken breast, turkey, tuna, salmon, beef) 2 cups of broccoli lightly stemmed (24 grams of carbs) or 2 bunch of broccoli rabe or 2 cups of brussel sprouts.

Snack
¼ cup of cottage cheese with ¼ of blueberries (7 grams of carbs) or 2 scoops of protein pudding

Water
_____12ounces		_____12ounces	
_____12ounces		_____12ounces	
_____12ounces		_____12ounces	
_____12ounces		_____12ounces	

The Low T Book Strength Training Exercise

Reverse Dumbbell Lunges

Set 1_____, Set 2 _____

Deep Knee Burlesque Squats

Set 1_____, Set 2 _____

Dumbbell Stiff Leg Deadlift

Set 1_____, Set 2 _____

Dumbbell Step Ups

Set 1_____, Set 2 _____

Squat and Press

Set 1_____, Set 2 _____

Incline Dumbbell Press

Set 1_____, Set 2 _____

Abdominal Wheel Rollouts

Set 1_____, Set 2 _____

Perform 2 sets of these exercises.

Set 1: 13-18 reps,

Set 2: 13-18 reps. <30 seconds rest between sets and 60 seconds rest between exercises.

Choose a weight that is 40-65% of your one rep max weight with proper form.

Fat Burning Finishing Exercise

Ski Jump-perform 4 sets of 25 reps

Set 1_____, Set 2 _____, Set 3_____, Set 4_____

Day 19-The Low T Book Aerobic Day Meals

Meal 1
Oatmeal Protein Pancakes:
2 scoops of protein powder mixed with ¾ cup of egg whites, ¼ teaspoon of cinnamon, one tablespoon of oats (10 grams). Add enough water for batter type consistency, spray skillet with cooking spray. Top with sugar free syrup or butter. (10 grams of carbs). 1/2 cup of strawberries (6 grams of carbs)

Snack
5.3-ounce container of plain Greek yogurt with ¼ cup of added fruit (10 grams of carbs) or 2 scoops of protein pudding

Meal 2
4-6 ounces of a lean protein (chicken breast, turkey, tuna, salmon, beef) on a bed of 2 cups of mixed leaf lettuces or spinach or romaine lettuce (2 grams of carbs) with a teaspoon of extra virgin olive oil and fresh lemon squeezed or 1 tbsp. of apple cider vinegar

Snack
15 raw almonds or walnuts (4 grams of carbs)

Meal 3
4-6 ounces of a lean protein (chicken breast, turkey, tuna, salmon, beef) 2 cups of cauliflower lightly stemmed and mashed with ½ teaspoon of olive oil (12 grams of carbs) or 12 asparagus spears.

Snack
¼ cup of cottage cheese with ¼ of strawberries (3 grams of carbs) or 2 scoops of protein pudding

Water
_____12ounces		_____12ounces	
_____12ounces		_____12ounces	
_____12ounces		_____12ounces	
_____12ounces		_____12ounces	

The Low T Book Guide Cardiovascular Exercise

1st Machine for 10-minutes

10 minutes warm up at 50% effort

2nd Machine for 10 minutes

1:30 seconds @ 50% effort
30 seconds @ 90% effort
1:30 seconds @ 50% effort
30 seconds @ 90% effort
1:30 seconds @ 50% effort
30 seconds @ 90% effort
1:30 seconds @ 50% effort
30 seconds @ 90% effort
1:30 seconds @ 50% effort
30 seconds @ 90% effort

REST FOR 3-5 MINUTES AND DRINK 6-8 0UNZES OF COLD WATER

3rd Machine for 10-20 minutes

10-20 minutes at 50% effort

Day 18- The Low T Book Strength Training Day Meals

Meal 1
Two large organic eggs with ½ cup of egg whites scrambled and one diced pepper, 1 tsp of crushed red pepper on a bed of 2 cups of spinach or arugula 2 slices of multigrain toast with butter (22 grams of carbs)
1 cup of halved strawberries (12 grams of carbs)

Snack
1 medium apple (20 grams of carbs) and 2 scoops of protein pudding

Meal 2
4-6 ounces of a lean protein (chicken breast, turkey, tuna, salmon, beef) on a bed of 2 cups of mixed leaf lettuces or spinach or romaine lettuce (2 grams of carbs) with a teaspoon of extra virgin olive oil and fresh lemon squeezed or 1 tbsp. of apple cider vinegar
1 medium apple (20 grams of carbs) or half a sweet potato

Snack
15 raw almonds or walnuts (4 grams of carbs)

Meal 3
4-6 ounces of a lean protein (chicken breast, turkey, tuna, salmon, beef)
2 cups of broccoli lightly stemmed (24 grams of carbs) or 2 bunch of broccoli rabe or 2 cups of brussel sprouts.

Snack
¼ cup of cottage cheese with ¼ of blueberries (7 grams of carbs) or 2 scoops of protein pudding

Water
_____12ounces	_____12ounces
_____12ounces	_____12ounces
_____12ounces	_____12ounces
_____12ounces	_____12ounces

The Low T Book Strength Training Exercise

Front Dumbbell Raises

Set 1_____, Set 2 _____

2 point Dumbbell Row

Set 1_____, Set 2 _____

Wide Hand Push ups

Set 1_____, Set 2 _____

Standing Dumbbell One Arm Triceps Extensions

Set 1_____, Set 2 _____

Standing Shoulder Press

Set 1_____, Set 2 _____

Dumbbell Triceps Kickback

Set 1_____, Set 2 _____

Plank

30 secs_____, 30 secs_____, 30 secs_____, 30 secs_____, 30 secs_____, 30 secs_____

Fat Burning Finishing Exercise:

Ski Jump-perform 4 sets of 25 reps

Set 1_____, Set 2 _____, Set 3_____, Set 4_____

Perform 2 sets of these exercises.

Set 1: 13-18 reps

Set 2: 13-18 reps. <30 seconds rest between sets and 60 seconds rest between exercises.

Choose a weight that is 40-65% of your one rep max weight with proper form.

Day 17-The Low T Book Aerobic Day Meals

Meal 1
Protein shake
½ cup of organic lactose free milk (7 grams of carbs)
1 scoop of protein powder (4 grams of carbs)
½ cup of blueberries or ½ cup of strawberries (10 grams of carbs)
¼ teaspoon of cinnamon
Add 1 cup of water, 3-5 ice cubes and blend in mixer

Snack
5.3-ounce container of plain Greek yogurt with ¼ cup of added fruit (10 grams of carbs) or 2 scoops of protein pudding

Meal 2
4-6 ounces of a lean protein (chicken breast, turkey, tuna, salmon, beef) on a bed of 2 cups of mixed leaf lettuces or spinach or romaine lettuce (2 grams of carbs) with a teaspoon of extra virgin olive oil and fresh lemon squeezed or 1 tbsp. of apple cider vinegar

Snack
15 raw almonds or walnuts (4 grams of carbs)

Meal 3
4-6 ounces of a lean protein (chicken breast, turkey, tuna, salmon, beef) 2 cups of cauliflower lightly stemmed and mashed with ½ teaspoon of olive oil (12 grams of carbs) or 12 asparagus spears.

Snack
¼ cup of cottage cheese with ¼ of strawberries (3 grams of carbs) or 2 scoops of protein pudding

Water
_____12ounces   _____12ounces
_____12ounces   _____12ounces
_____12ounces   _____12ounces
_____12ounces   _____12ounces

The Low T Book Guide Cardiovascular Exercise

1st Machine for 10-minutes

10 minutes warm up at 50% effort

2nd Machine for 10 minutes

1:30 seconds @ 50% effort
30 seconds @ 90% effort
1:30 seconds @ 50% effort
30 seconds @ 90% effort
1:30 seconds @ 50% effort
30 seconds @ 90% effort
1:30 seconds @ 50% effort
30 seconds @ 90% effort
1:30 seconds @ 50% effort
30 seconds @ 90% effort

REST FOR 3-5 MINUTES AND DRINK 6-8 0UNZES OF COLD WATER

3rd Machine for 10-20 minutes

10-20 minutes at 50% effort

Day 16- The Low T Book Strength Training Day Meals

Meal 1
Two large organic eggs with ½ cup of egg whites scrambled and one diced pepper, 1 tsp of crushed red pepper on a bed of 2 cups of spinach or arugula 2 slices of multigrain toast with butter (22 grams of carbs) 1 cup of halved strawberries (12 grams of carbs)

Snack
1 medium apple (20 grams of carbs) and 2 scoops of protein pudding

Meal 2
4-6 ounces of a lean protein (chicken breast, turkey, tuna, salmon, beef) on a bed of 2 cups of mixed leaf lettuces or spinach or romaine lettuce (2 grams of carbs) with a teaspoon of extra virgin olive oil and fresh lemon squeezed or 1 tbsp. of apple cider vinegar
1 medium apple (20 grams of carbs) or half a sweet potato

Snack
15 raw almonds or walnuts (4 grams of carbs)

Meal 3
4-6 ounces of a lean protein (chicken breast, turkey, tuna, salmon, beef)
2 cups of broccoli lightly stemmed (24 grams of carbs) or 2 bunch of broccoli rabe or 2 cups of brussel sprouts.

Snack
¼ cup of cottage cheese with ¼ of blueberries (7 grams of carbs) or 2 scoops of protein pudding

Water

_____12ounces		_____12ounces	
_____12ounces		_____12ounces	
_____12ounces		_____12ounces	
_____12ounces		_____12ounces	

The Low T Book Strength Training Exercise

Heart to Heart Pushup

Set 1_____, Set 2 _____

Dumbbell Stiff Leg Deadlift

Set 1_____, Set 2 _____

Dumbbell Step Ups

Set 1_____, Set 2 _____

Squat and Press

Set 1_____, Set 2 _____

Incline Dumbbell Press

Set 1_____, Set 2 _____

Bent Lateral Raises

Set 1_____, Set 2 _____

Abdominal Wheel Rollouts

Set 1_____, Set 2 _____

Fat Burning Finishing Exercise:

Squat and Thrust-perform 4 sets of 25 reps

Set 1_____, Set 2 _____, Set 3_____, Set 4____

Perform 2 sets of these exercises.

Set 1: 13-18 reps

Set 2: 13-18 reps. <30 seconds rest between sets and 60 seconds rest between exercises.

Choose a weight that is 40-65% of your one rep max weight with proper form.

Day 15- The Low T Book Aerobic Day Meals

Meal 1
Oatmeal Protein Pancakes:
2 scoops of protein powder mixed with ¾ cup of egg whites, ¼ teaspoon of cinnamon, one tablespoon of oats (10 grams). Add enough water for batter type consistency, spray skillet with cooking spray. Top with sugar free syrup or butter. (10 grams of carbs). 1/2 cup of strawberries (6 grams of carbs)

Snack
5.3-ounce container of plain Greek yogurt with ¼ cup of added fruit (10 grams of carbs) or 2 scoops of protein pudding

Meal 2
4-6 ounces of a lean protein (chicken breast, turkey, tuna, salmon, beef) on a bed of 2 cups of mixed leaf lettuces or spinach or romaine lettuce (2 grams of carbs) with a teaspoon of extra virgin olive oil and fresh lemon squeezed or 1 tbsp. of apple cider vinegar
Snack
15 raw almonds or walnuts (4 grams of carbs)

Meal 3
4-6 ounces of a lean protein (chicken breast, turkey, tuna, salmon, beef) 2 cups of cauliflower lightly stemmed and mashed with ½ teaspoon of olive oil (12 grams of carbs) or 12 asparagus spears.

Snack
¼ cup of cottage cheese with ¼ of strawberries (3 grams of carbs) or 2 scoops of protein pudding

Water
_____12ounces		_____12ounces	
_____12ounces		_____12ounces	
_____12ounces		_____12ounces	
_____12ounces		_____12ounces	

The Low T Book Guide Cardiovascular Exercise

1st Machine for 10-minutes

10 minutes warm up at 50% effort

2nd Machine for 10 minutes

1:30 seconds @ 50% effort
30 seconds @ 90% effort
1:30 seconds @ 50% effort
30 seconds @ 90% effort
1:30 seconds @ 50% effort
30 seconds @ 90% effort
1:30 seconds @ 50% effort
30 seconds @ 90% effort
1:30 seconds @ 50% effort
30 seconds @ 90% effort

REST FOR 3-5 MINUTES AND DRINK 6-8 0UNZES OF COLD WATER

3rd Machine for 10-20 minutes

10-20 minutes at 50% effort

Day 14- The Low T Book Strength Training Day Meals

Meal 1
Two large organic eggs with ½ cup of egg whites scrambled and one diced pepper, 1 tsp of crushed red pepper on a bed of 2 cups of spinach or arugula 2 slices of multigrain toast with butter (22 grams of carbs)
1 cup of halved strawberries (12 grams of carbs)

Snack
1 medium apple (20 grams of carbs) and 2 scoops of protein pudding

Meal 2
4-6 ounces of a lean protein (chicken breast, turkey, tuna, salmon, beef) on a bed of 2 cups of mixed leaf lettuces or spinach or romaine lettuce (2 grams of carbs) with a teaspoon of extra virgin olive oil and fresh lemon squeezed or 1 tbsp. of apple cider vinegar
1 medium apple (20 grams of carbs) or half a sweet potato

Snack
15 raw almonds or walnuts (4 grams of carbs)

Meal 3
4-6 ounces of a lean protein (chicken breast, turkey, tuna, salmon, beef)
2 cups of broccoli lightly stemmed (24 grams of carbs) or 2 bunch of broccoli rabe or 2 cups of brussel sprouts.

Snack
¼ cup of cottage cheese with ¼ of blueberries (7 grams of carbs) or 2 scoops of protein pudding

Water
_____12ounces		_____12ounces	
_____12ounces		_____12ounces	
_____12ounces		_____12ounces	
_____12ounces		_____12ounces	

The Low T Book Strength Training Exercise

Dumbbell Hammer Curls

Set 1_____, Set 2 _____

Standing Dumbbell Concentration Curls

Set 1_____, Set 2 _____

Seated Shoulder press

Set 1_____, Set 2 _____

2 point Dumbbell Row

Set 1_____, Set 2 _____

Dumbbell Front Raise

Set 1_____, Set 2 _____

Bent Dumbbell Lateral Raises

Set 1_____, Set 2 _____

Plank

30 secs_____, 30 secs_____, 30 secs_____, 30 secs_____, 30 secs_____,
30 secs_____

Perform 2 sets of these exercises.

Set 1: 13-18 reps

Set 2: 13-18 reps. <30 seconds rest between sets and 60 seconds rest between exercises.

Choose a weight that is 40-65% of your one rep max weight with proper form.

Fat Burning Finishing Exercise:

Squat and Thrust-perform 4 sets of 25 reps

Set 1_____, Set 2 _____, Set 3_____, Set 4____

Day 13- The Low T Book Aerobic Day Meals /Optional Exercise OFF Day

Meal 1
Protein shake
½ cup of organic lactose free milk (7 grams of carbs)
1 scoop of protein powder (4 grams of carbs)
½ cup of blueberries or ½ cup of strawberries (10 grams of carbs)
¼ teaspoon of cinnamon
Add 1 cup of water, 3-5 ice cubes and blend in mixer

Snack
5.3-ounce container of plain Greek yogurt with ¼ cup of added fruit (10 grams of carbs) or 2 scoops of protein pudding

Meal 2
4-6 ounces of a lean protein (chicken breast, turkey, tuna, salmon, beef) on a bed of 2 cups of mixed leaf lettuces or spinach or romaine lettuce (2 grams of carbs) with a teaspoon of extra virgin olive oil and fresh lemon squeezed or 1 tbsp. of apple cider vinegar

Snack
15 raw almonds or walnuts (4 grams of carbs)

Meal 3
4-6 ounces of a lean protein (chicken breast, turkey, tuna, salmon, beef) 2 cups of cauliflower lightly stemmed and mashed with ½ teaspoon of olive oil (12 grams of carbs) or 12 asparagus spears.

Snack
¼ cup of cottage cheese with ¼ of strawberries (3 grams of carbs) or 2 scoops of protein pudding

Water
_____12ounces _____12ounces
_____12ounces _____12ounces
_____12ounces _____12ounces
_____12ounces _____12ounces

The Low T Book Guide Cardiovascular Exercise

1st Machine for 10-minutes

10 minutes warm up at 50% effort

2nd Machine for 10 minutes

1:30 seconds @ 50% effort
30 seconds @ 90% effort
1:30 seconds @ 50% effort
30 seconds @ 90% effort
1:30 seconds @ 50% effort
30 seconds @ 90% effort
1:30 seconds @ 50% effort
30 seconds @ 90% effort
1:30 seconds @ 50% effort
30 seconds @ 90% effort

REST FOR 3-5 MINUTES AND DRINK 6-8 0UNZES OF COLD WATER

3rd Machine for 10-20 minutes

10-20 minutes at 50% effort

Day 12- The Low T Book Strength Training Day Meals

Meal 1
Two large organic eggs with ½ cup of egg whites scrambled and one diced pepper, 1 tsp of crushed red pepper on a bed of 2 cups of spinach or arugula 2 slices of multigrain toast with butter (22 grams of carbs) 1 cup of halved strawberries (12 grams of carbs)

Snack
1 medium apple (20 grams of carbs) and 2 scoops of protein pudding

Meal 2
4-6 ounces of a lean protein (chicken breast, turkey, tuna, salmon, beef) on a bed of 2 cups of mixed leaf lettuces or spinach or romaine lettuce (2 grams of carbs) with a teaspoon of extra virgin olive oil and fresh lemon squeezed or 1 tbsp. of apple cider vinegar
1 medium apple (20 grams of carbs) or half a sweet potato

Snack
15 raw almonds or walnuts (4 grams of carbs)

Meal 3
4-6 ounces of a lean protein (chicken breast, turkey, tuna, salmon, beef) 2 cups of broccoli lightly stemmed (24 grams of carbs) or 2 bunch of broccoli rabe or 2 cups of brussel sprouts.

Snack
¼ cup of cottage cheese with ¼ of blueberries (7 grams of carbs) or 2 scoops of protein pudding

Water
_____12ounces	_____12ounces
_____12ounces	_____12ounces
_____12ounces	_____12ounces
_____12ounces	_____12ounces

The Low T Book Strength Training Exercise

Deep Knee Burlesque Squats

Set 1_____, Set 2 _____

Reverse Dumbbell Lunges

Set 1_____, Set 2 _____

Dumbbell Step Ups

Set 1_____, Set 2 _____

Incline Dumbbell Press

Set 1_____, Set 2 _____

Curl and Press

Set 1_____, Set 2 _____

Front Dumbbell Raises

Set 1_____, Set 2 _____

Abdominal Wheel Rollouts

Set 1_____, Set 2 _____

Perform 2 sets of these exercises.

Set 1: 13-18 reps

Set 2: 13-18 reps. <30 seconds rest between sets and 60 seconds rest between exercises.

Choose a weight that is 40-65% of your one rep max weight with proper form.

Fat Burning Finishing Exercise:

Squat and Thrust-perform 4 sets of 25 reps

Set 1_____, Set 2 _____, Set 3_____, Set 4____

Day 11- The Low T Book Aerobic Day Meals

Meal 1
Oatmeal Protein Pancakes:
2 scoops of protein powder mixed with ¾ cup of egg whites, ¼ teaspoon of cinnamon, one tablespoon of oats (10 grams). Add enough water for batter type consistency, spray skillet with cooking spray. Top with sugar free syrup or butter. (10 grams of carbs). 1/2 cup of strawberries (6 grams of carbs)

Snack
5.3-ounce container of plain Greek yogurt with ¼ cup of added fruit (10 grams of carbs) or 2 scoops of protein pudding

Meal 2
4-6 ounces of a lean protein (chicken breast, turkey, tuna, salmon, beef) on a bed of 2 cups of mixed leaf lettuces or spinach or romaine lettuce (2 grams of carbs) with a teaspoon of extra virgin olive oil and fresh lemon squeezed or 1 tbsp. of apple cider vinegar

Snack
15 raw almonds or walnuts (4 grams of carbs)

Meal 3
4-6 ounces of a lean protein (chicken breast, turkey, tuna, salmon, beef) 2 cups of cauliflower lightly stemmed and mashed with ½ teaspoon of olive oil (12 grams of carbs) or 12 asparagus spears.

Snack
¼ cup of cottage cheese with ¼ of blueberries (7 grams of carbs) or 2 scoops of protein pudding

Water
_____12ounces   _____12ounces
_____12ounces   _____12ounces
_____12ounces   _____12ounces
_____12ounces   _____12ounces

The Low T Book Guide Cardiovascular Exercise

1st Machine for 10-minutes

10 minutes warm up at 50% effort

2nd Machine for 10 minutes

1:30 seconds @ 50% effort
30 seconds @ 90% effort
1:30 seconds @ 50% effort
30 seconds @ 90% effort
1:30 seconds @ 50% effort
30 seconds @ 90% effort
1:30 seconds @ 50% effort
30 seconds @ 90% effort
1:30 seconds @ 50% effort
30 seconds @ 90% effort

REST FOR 3-5 MINUTES AND DRINK 6-8 0UNZES OF COLD WATER

3rd Machine for 10-20 minutes

10-20 minutes at 50% effort

Day 10- The Low T Book Strength Training Day Meals

Meal 1
Two large organic eggs with ½ cup of egg whites scrambled and one diced pepper, 1 tsp of crushed red pepper on a bed of 2 cups of spinach or arugula 2 slices of multigrain toast with butter (22 grams of carbs)
1 cup of halved strawberries (12 grams of carbs)

Snack
1 medium apple (20 grams of carbs) and 2 scoops of protein pudding

Meal 2
4-6 ounces of a lean protein (chicken breast, turkey, tuna, salmon, beef) on a bed of 2 cups of mixed leaf lettuces or spinach or romaine lettuce (2 grams of carbs) with a teaspoon of extra virgin olive oil and fresh lemon squeezed or 1 tbsp. of apple cider vinegar
1 medium apple (20 grams of carbs) or half a sweet potato

Snack
15 raw almonds or walnuts (4 grams of carbs)

Meal 3
4-6 ounces of a lean protein (chicken breast, turkey, tuna, salmon, beef) 2 cups of broccoli lightly stemmed (24 grams of carbs) or 2 bunch of broccoli rabe or 2 cups of brussel sprouts.

Snack
¼ cup of cottage cheese with ¼ of blueberries (7 grams of carbs) or 2 scoops of protein pudding

Water
_____12ounces	_____12ounces
_____12ounces	_____12ounces
_____12ounces	_____12ounces
_____12ounces	_____12ounces

The Low T Book Strength Training Exercise

Wide Hand Push Ups

Set 1_____, Set 2 _____

Incline Triceps Extensions

Set 1_____, Set 2 _____

Heart to Heart Push Ups

Set 1_____, Set 2 _____

Dumbbell Triceps Kickback

Set 1_____, Set 2 _____

Seated Dumbbell Shoulder Press

Set 1_____, Set 2 _____

Dumbbell Upright Row

Set 1_____, Set 2 _____

Plank

30 secs_____, 30 secs_____, 30 secs_____, 30 secs_____, 30 secs_____, 30 secs_____

Perform 2 sets of these exercises.

Set 1: 13-18 reps

Set 2: 13-18 reps. <30 seconds rest between sets and 60 seconds rest between exercises.

Choose a weight that is 40-65% of your one rep max weight with proper form.

Fat Burning Finishing Exercise:

Ski Jump-perform 4 sets of 25 reps

Set 1_____, Set 2 _____, Set 3_____, Set 4_____

Day 9- The Low T Book Aerobic Day Meals

Meal 1
Protein shake
½ cup of organic lactose free milk (7 grams of carbs)
1 scoop of protein powder (4 grams of carbs)
½ cup of blueberries or ½ cup of strawberries (10 grams of carbs)
¼ teaspoon of cinnamon
1 cup of water, 3-5 ice cubes and blend in mixer

Snack
5.3-ounce container of plain Greek yogurt with ¼ cup of added fruit (10 grams of carbs) or 2 scoops of protein pudding

Meal 2
4-6 ounces of a lean protein (chicken breast, turkey, tuna, salmon, beef) on a bed of 2 cups of mixed leaf lettuces or spinach or romaine lettuce (2 grams of carbs) with a teaspoon of extra virgin olive oil and fresh lemon squeezed or 1 tbsp. of apple cider vinegar

Snack
15 raw almonds or walnuts (4 grams of carbs)

Meal 3
4-6 ounces of a lean protein (chicken breast, turkey, tuna, salmon, beef) 2 cups of cauliflower lightly stemmed and mashed with ½ teaspoon of olive oil (12 grams of carbs) or 12 asparagus spears.

Snack
¼ cup of cottage cheese with ¼ of blueberries (7 grams of carbs) or 2 scoops of protein pudding

Water
_____12ounces		_____12ounces	
_____12ounces		_____12ounces	
_____12ounces		_____12ounces	
_____12ounces		_____12ounces	

The Low T Book Guide Cardiovascular Exercise

1st Machine for 10-minutes

10 minutes warm up at 50% effort

2nd Machine for 10 minutes

1:30 seconds @ 50% effort
30 seconds @ 90% effort
1:30 seconds @ 50% effort
30 seconds @ 90% effort
1:30 seconds @ 50% effort
30 seconds @ 90% effort
1:30 seconds @ 50% effort
30 seconds @ 90% effort
1:30 seconds @ 50% effort
30 seconds @ 90% effort

REST FOR 3-5 MINUTES AND DRINK 6-8 0UNZES OF COLD WATER

3rd Machine for 10-20 minutes

10-20 minutes at 50% effort

Day 8- The Low T Book Strength Training Day Meals

Meal 1
Two large organic eggs with ½ cup of egg whites scrambled and one diced pepper, 1 tsp of crushed red pepper on a bed of 2 cups of spinach or arugula 2 slices of multigrain toast with butter (22 grams of carbs) 1 cup of halved strawberries (12 grams of carbs)

Snack
1 medium apple (20 grams of carbs) and 2 scoops of protein pudding

Meal 2
4-6 ounces of a lean protein (chicken breast, turkey, tuna, salmon, beef) on a bed of 2 cups of mixed leaf lettuces or spinach or romaine lettuce (2 grams of carbs) with a teaspoon of extra virgin olive oil and fresh lemon squeezed or 1 tbsp. of apple cider vinegar
1 medium apple (20 grams of carbs) or half a sweet potato

Snack
15 raw almonds or walnuts (4 grams of carbs)

Meal 3
4-6 ounces of a lean protein (chicken breast, turkey, tuna, salmon, beef) 2 cups of broccoli lightly stemmed (24 grams of carbs) or 2 bunch of broccoli rabe or 2 cups of brussel sprouts.

Snack
¼ cup of cottage cheese with ¼ of blueberries (7 grams of carbs) or 2 scoops of protein pudding

Water
_____12ounces		_____12ounces	
_____12ounces		_____12ounces	
_____12ounces		_____12ounces	
_____12ounces		_____12ounces	

The Low T Book Strength Training Exercise

One Leg Calf raises

Set 1_____, Set 2 _____

Incline Dumbbell Fly

Set 1_____, Set 2 _____

Dumbbell Lateral Raises

Set 1_____, Set 2 _____

Alternating Incline Dumbbell Press

Set 1_____, Set 2 _____

Standing Dumbbell Shoulder Press

Set 1_____, Set 2 _____

Dumbbell Front Raises

Set 1_____, Set 2 _____

Abdominal Wheel Rollouts

Set 1_____, Set 2 _____

Perform 2 sets of these exercises.

Set 1: 13-18 reps

Set 2: 13-18 reps. <30 seconds rest between sets and 60 seconds rest between exercises.

Choose a weight that is 40-65% of your one rep max weight with proper form.

Fat Burning Finishing Exercise:

Squat and Thrust-perform 4 sets of 25 reps

Set 1_____, Set 2 _____, Set 3_____, Set 4____

Day 7- The Low T Book Aerobic Day Meals

Meal 1
Oatmeal Protein Pancakes:
2 scoops of protein powder mixed with ¾ cup of egg whites, ¼ teaspoon of cinnamon, one tablespoon of oats (10 grams). Add enough water for batter type consistency, spray skillet with cooking spray. Top with sugar free syrup or butter. (10 grams of carbs). 1/2 cup of strawberries (6 grams of carbs)

Snack
5.3-ounce container of plain Greek yogurt with ¼ cup of added fruit (10 grams of carbs) or 2 scoops of protein pudding

Meal 2
4-6 ounces of a lean protein (chicken breast, turkey, tuna, salmon, beef) on a bed of 2 cups mixed leaf lettuces or spinach or romaine lettuce (2 grams of carbs) with a teaspoon of extra virgin olive oil and fresh lemon squeezed

Snack
15 raw almonds or walnuts (4 grams of carbs)

Meal 3
4-6 ounces of a lean protein (chicken breast, turkey, tuna, salmon, beef) 2 cups of cauliflower lightly stemmed and mashed with ½ teaspoon of olive oil (12 grams of carbs) or 12 asparagus spears.

Snack
¼ cup of cottage cheese with ¼ of blueberries (7 grams of carbs) or 2 scoops of protein pudding

Water
_____12ounces	_____12ounces	
_____12ounces	_____12ounces	
_____12ounces	_____12ounces	
_____12ounces	_____12ounces	

The Low T Book Guide Cardiovascular Exercise

1st Machine for 10-minutes

10 minutes warm up at 50% effort

2nd Machine for 10 minutes

1:30 seconds @ 50% effort
30 seconds @ 90% effort
1:30 seconds @ 50% effort
30 seconds @ 90% effort
1:30 seconds @ 50% effort
30 seconds @ 90% effort
1:30 seconds @ 50% effort
30 seconds @ 90% effort
1:30 seconds @ 50% effort
30 seconds @ 90% effort

REST FOR 3-5 MINUTES AND DRINK 6-8 0UNZES OF COLD WATER

3rd Machine for 10-20 minutes

10-20 minutes at 50% effort

Day 6- The Low T Book Strength Training Day Meals

Meal 1
Two large organic eggs with ½ cup of egg whites scrambled and one diced pepper, 1 tsp of crushed red pepper on a bed of 2 cups of spinach or arugula 2 slices of multigrain toast with butter (22 grams of carbs)
1 cup of halved strawberries (12 grams of carbs)

Snack
1 medium apple (20 grams of carbs) and 2 scoops of protein pudding

Meal 2
4-6 ounces of a lean protein (chicken breast, turkey, tuna, salmon, beef) on a bed of 2 cups of mixed leaf lettuces or spinach or romaine lettuce (2 grams of carbs) with a teaspoon of extra virgin olive oil and fresh lemon squeezed or 1 tbsp. of apple cider vinegar
1 medium apple (20 grams of carbs) or half a sweet potato

Snack
15 raw almonds or walnuts (4 grams of carbs)

Meal 3
4-6 ounces of a lean protein (chicken breast, turkey, tuna, salmon, beef)
2 cups of broccoli lightly stemmed (24 grams of carbs) or 2 bunch of broccoli rabe or 2 cups of brussel sprouts.

Snack
¼ cup of cottage cheese with ¼ of blueberries (7 grams of carbs) or 2 scoops of protein pudding

Water
_____12ounces		_____12ounces	
_____12ounces		_____12ounces	
_____12ounces		_____12ounces	
_____12ounces		_____12ounces	

The Low T Book Strength Training Exercise

Dumbbell Bench Step Ups

Set 1_____, Set 2 _____

Plank Alternating Knee to Elbow

Set 1_____, Set 2 _____

Dumbbell Triceps Kickbacks

Set 1_____, Set 2 _____

Bent Dumbbell Face Row

Set 1_____, Set 2 _____

Flat Dumbbell Press

Set 1_____, Set 2 _____

Standing Dumbbell Lateral Raises
Set 1_____, Set 2 _____

Plank

30 secs_____, 30 secs_____, 30 secs_____, 30 secs_____, 30 secs_____,
30 secs_____

Perform 2 sets of these exercises.

Set 1: 13-18 reps

Set 2: 13-18 reps. <30 seconds rest between sets and 60 seconds rest between exercises.

Choose a weight that is 40-65% of your one rep max weight with proper form.

Fat Burning Finishing Exercise:

Squat and Thrust-perform 4 sets of 25 reps

Set 1_____, Set 2 _____, Set 3_____, Set 4____

Day 5- The Low T Book Aerobic Day Meals /Optional Exercise OFF Day

Meal 1
Protein shake
½ cup of organic lactose free milk (7 grams of carbs)
1 scoop of protein powder (4 grams of carbs)
½ cup of blueberries or ½ cup of strawberries (10 grams of carbs)
¼ teaspoon of cinnamon
Add 1 cup of water, 3-5 ice cubes and blend in mixer

Snack
5.3-ounce container of plain Greek yogurt with ¼ cup of added fruit (10 grams of carbs) or 2 scoops of protein pudding

Meal 2
4-6 ounces of a lean protein (chicken breast, turkey, tuna, salmon, beef) on a bed of 2 cups of mixed leaf lettuces or spinach or romaine lettuce (2 grams of carbs) with a teaspoon of extra virgin olive oil and fresh lemon squeezed or 1 tbsp. of apple cider vinegar

Snack
15 raw almonds or walnuts (4 grams of carbs)

Meal 3
4-6 ounces of a lean protein (chicken breast, turkey, tuna, salmon, beef) 2 cups of cauliflower lightly stemmed and mashed with ½ teaspoon of olive oil (12 grams of carbs) or 12 asparagus spears.

Snack
¼ cup of cottage cheese with ¼ of blueberries (7 grams of carbs) or 2 scoops of protein pudding

Water
_____12ounces   _____12ounces
_____12ounces   _____12ounces
_____12ounces   _____12ounces
_____12ounces   _____12ounces

The Low T Book Guide Cardiovascular Exercise

1st Machine for 10-minutes

10 minutes warm up at 50% effort

2nd Machine for 10 minutes

1:30 seconds @ 50% effort
30 seconds @ 90% effort
1:30 seconds @ 50% effort
30 seconds @ 90% effort
1:30 seconds @ 50% effort
30 seconds @ 90% effort
1:30 seconds @ 50% effort
30 seconds @ 90% effort
1:30 seconds @ 50% effort
30 seconds @ 90% effort

REST FOR 3-5 MINUTES AND DRINK 6-8 0UNZES OF COLD WATER

3rd Machine for 10-20 minutes

10-20 minutes at 50% effort

Day 4- The Low T Book Strength Training Day Meals

Meal 1
Two large organic eggs with ½ cup of egg whites scrambled and one diced pepper, 1 tsp of crushed red pepper on a bed of 2 cups of spinach or arugula 2 slices of multigrain toast with butter (22 grams of carbs) 1 cup of halved strawberries (12 grams of carbs)

Snack
1 medium apple (20 grams of carbs) and 2 scoops of protein pudding

Meal 2
4-6 ounces of a lean protein (chicken breast, turkey, tuna, salmon, beef) on a bed of 2 cups of mixed leaf lettuces or spinach or romaine lettuce (2 grams of carbs) with a teaspoon of extra virgin olive oil and fresh lemon squeezed or 1 tbsp. of apple cider vinegar
1 medium apple (20 grams of carbs) or half a sweet potato

Snack
15 raw almonds or walnuts (4 grams of carbs)

Meal 3
4-6 ounces of a lean protein (chicken breast, turkey, tuna, salmon, beef) 2 cups of broccoli lightly stemmed (24 grams of carbs) or 2 bunch of broccoli rabe or 2 cups of brussel sprouts.

Snack
¼ cup of cottage cheese with ¼ of blueberries (7 grams of carbs) or 2 scoops of protein pudding

Water
_____12ounces		_____12ounces	
_____12ounces		_____12ounces	
_____12ounces		_____12ounces	
_____12ounces		_____12ounces	

The Low T Book Strength Training Exercise

Dumbbell Bench Step Ups

Set 1_____, Set 2 _____

Deep Knee Burlesque Squats

Set 1_____, Set 2 _____

Dumbbell Straight Leg Deadlift

Set 1_____, Set 2 _____

Dumbbell Reverse Lunge

Set 1_____, Set 2 _____

Incline Dumbbell Press

Set 1_____, Set 2 _____

Dumbbell Forward Lunge

Set 1_____, Set 2 _____

Front Dumbbell Raise

Set 1_____, Set 2 _____

Perform 2 sets of these exercises.

Set 1:13-18 reps

Set 2:13-18 reps. <30 seconds rest between sets and 60 seconds rest between exercises.

Choose a weight that is 40-65% of your one rep max weight with proper form.

Fat Burning Finishing Exercise:

Squat and Thrust-perform 4 sets of 25 reps

Set 1_____, Set 2 _____, Set 3_____, Set 4____

Day 3- The Low T Book Aerobic Day Meals

Meal 1
Oatmeal Protein Pancakes:
2 scoops of protein powder mixed with ¾ cup of egg whites, ¼ teaspoon of cinnamon, one tablespoon of oats (10 grams). Add enough water for batter type consistency, spray skillet with cooking spray. Top with sugar free syrup or butter. (10 grams of carbs). 1/2 cup of strawberries (6 grams of carbs)

Snack
5.3-ounce container of plain Greek yogurt with ¼ cup of added fruit (10 grams of carbs) or 2 scoops of protein pudding

Meal 2
4-6 ounces of a lean protein (chicken breast, turkey, tuna, salmon, beef) on a bed of 2 cups of mixed leaf lettuces or spinach or romaine lettuce (2 grams of carbs) with a teaspoon of extra virgin olive oil and fresh lemon squeezed or 1 tbsp. of apple cider vinegar

Snack
15 raw almonds or walnuts (4 grams of carbs)

Meal 3
4-6 ounces of a lean protein (chicken breast, turkey, tuna, salmon, beef) 2 cups of cauliflower lightly stemmed and mashed with ½ teaspoon of olive oil (12 grams of carbs) or 12 asparagus spears.

Snack
¼ cup of cottage cheese with ¼ of blueberries (7 grams of carbs) or 2 scoops of protein pudding

Water
_____12ounces   _____12ounces
_____12ounces   _____12ounces
_____12ounces   _____12ounces
_____12ounces   _____12ounces

The Low T Book Guide Cardiovascular Exercise

1st Machine for 10-minutes

10 minutes warm up at 50% effort

2nd Machine for 10 minutes

1:30 seconds @ 50% effort
30 seconds @ 90% effort
1:30 seconds @ 50% effort
30 seconds @ 90% effort
1:30 seconds @ 50% effort
30 seconds @ 90% effort
1:30 seconds @ 50% effort
30 seconds @ 90% effort
1:30 seconds @ 50% effort
30 seconds @ 90% effort

REST FOR 3-5 MINUTES AND DRINK 6-8 0UNZES OF COLD WATER

3rd Machine for 10-20 minutes

10-20 minutes at 50% effort

Day 2- The Low T Book Strength Training Day Meals

Meal 1
Two large organic eggs with ½ cup of egg whites scrambled and one diced pepper, 1 tsp of crushed red pepper on a bed of 2 cups of spinach or arugula 2 slices of multigrain toast with butter (22 grams of carbs)
1 cup of halved strawberries (12 grams of carbs)

Snack
1 medium apple (20 grams of carbs) and 2 scoops of protein pudding

Meal 2
4-6 ounces of a lean protein (chicken breast, turkey, tuna, salmon, beef) on a bed of 2 cups of mixed leaf lettuces or spinach or romaine lettuce (2 grams of carbs) with a teaspoon of extra virgin olive oil and fresh lemon squeezed or 1 tbsp. of apple cider vinegar
1 medium apple (20 grams of carbs) or half a sweet potato

Snack
15 raw almonds or walnuts (4 grams of carbs)

Meal 3
4-6 ounces of a lean protein (chicken breast, turkey, tuna, salmon, beef)
2 cups of broccoli lightly stemmed (24 grams of carbs) or 2 bunch of broccoli rabe or 2 cups of brussel sprouts.

Snack
¼ cup of cottage cheese with ¼ of blueberries (7 grams of carbs) or 2 scoops of protein pudding

Water
_____12ounces		_____12ounces	
_____12ounces		_____12ounces	
_____12ounces		_____12ounces	
_____12ounces		_____12ounces	

The Low T Book Strength Training Exercise

Push Ups

Set 1_____, Set 2 _____

Dumbbell Single Leg Calf Raises

Set 1_____, Set 2 _____

Flat Dumbbell Press

Set 1_____, Set 2 _____

Dumbbell Upright Row

Set 1_____, Set 2 _____

Incline Dumbbell Press

Set 1_____, Set 2 _____

Standing Dumbbell Lateral Raise

Set 1_____, Set 2 _____

Plank

30 secs_____, 30 secs_____, 30 secs_____, 30 secs_____, 30 secs_____, 30 secs_____

Perform 2 sets of these exercises.

Set 1: 13-18 reps

Set 2: 13-18 reps. <30 seconds rest between sets and 60 seconds rest between exercises.

Choose a weight that is 40-65% of your one rep max weight with proper form.

Fat Burning Finishing Exercise:

Ski Jump-perform 4 sets of 25 reps

Set 1_____, Set 2 _____, Set 3_____, Set 4____

Day 1- The Low T Book Aerobic Day Meals

Meal 1
Protein shake
½ cup of organic lactose free milk (7 grams of carbs)
1 scoop of protein powder (4 grams of carbs)
½ cup of blueberries or ½ cup of strawberries (10 grams of carbs)
¼ teaspoon of cinnamon
Add 1 cup of water, 3-5 ice cubes and blend in mixer

Snack
5.3-ounce container of plain Greek yogurt with ¼ cup of added fruit (10 grams of carbs) or 2 scoops of protein pudding

Meal 2
4-6 ounces of a lean protein (chicken breast, turkey, tuna, salmon, beef) on a bed of 2 cups of mixed leaf lettuces or spinach or romaine lettuce (2 grams of carbs) with a teaspoon of extra virgin olive oil and fresh lemon squeezed or 1 tbsp. of apple cider vinegar

Snack
15 raw almonds or walnuts (4 grams of carbs)

Meal 3
4-6 ounces of a lean protein (chicken breast, turkey, tuna, salmon, beef) 2 cups of cauliflower lightly stemmed and mashed with ½ teaspoon of olive oil (12 grams of carbs) or 12 asparagus spears.

Snack
¼ cup of cottage cheese with ¼ of blueberries (7 grams of carbs) or 2 scoops of protein pudding

Water
_____12ounces   _____12ounces
_____12ounces   _____12ounces
_____12ounces   _____12ounces
_____12ounces   _____12ounces

The Low T Book Guide Cardiovascular Exercise

1st Machine for 10-minutes

10 minutes warm up at 50% effort

2nd Machine for 10 minutes

1:30 seconds @ 50% effort
30 seconds @ 90% effort
1:30 seconds @ 50% effort
30 seconds @ 90% effort
1:30 seconds @ 50% effort
30 seconds @ 90% effort
1:30 seconds @ 50% effort
30 seconds @ 90% effort
1:30 seconds @ 50% effort
30 seconds @ 90% effort

REST FOR 3-5 MINUTES AND DRINK 6-8 0UNZES OF COLD WATER

3rd Machine for 10-20 minutes

10-20 minutes at 50% effort

Day 0- The Low T Book Strength Training Day Meals

Meal 1
Two large organic eggs with ½ cup of egg whites scrambled and one diced pepper, 1 tsp of crushed red pepper on a bed of 2 cups of spinach or arugula 2 slices of multigrain toast with butter (22 grams of carbs) 1 cup of halved strawberries (12 grams of carbs)

Snack
1 medium apple (20 grams of carbs) and 2 scoops of protein pudding

Meal 2
4-6 ounces of a lean protein (chicken breast, turkey, tuna, salmon, beef) on a bed of 2 cups of mixed leaf lettuces or spinach or romaine lettuce (2 grams of carbs) with a teaspoon of extra virgin olive oil and fresh lemon squeezed or 1 tbsp. of apple cider vinegar
1 medium apple (20 grams of carbs) or half a sweet potato

Snack
15 raw almonds or walnuts (4 grams of carbs)

Meal 3
4-6 ounces of a lean protein (chicken breast, turkey, tuna, salmon, beef) 2 cups of broccoli lightly stemmed (24 grams of carbs) or 2 bunch of broccoli rabe or 2 cups of brussel sprouts.

Snack
¼ cup of cottage cheese with ¼ of blueberries (7 grams of carbs) or 2 scoops of protein pudding

Water
_____12ounces		_____12ounces
_____12ounces		_____12ounces
_____12ounces		_____12ounces
_____12ounces		_____12ounces

The Low T Book Strength Training Exercise

Seated Incline Dumbbell Curl

Set 1_____, Set 2 _____

Standing Dumbbell Curl

Set 1_____, Set 2 _____

Incline Dumbbell Fly

Set 1_____, Set 2 _____

Dumbbell Squat and Press

Set 1_____, Set 2 _____

Incline Dumbbell Press

Set 1_____, Set 2 _____

Dumbbell Front Raise

Set 1_____, Set 2 _____

Abdominal Wheel Rollouts

Set 1_____, Set 2 _____

Perform 2 sets of these exercises.

Set 1: 13-18 reps

Set 2: 13-18 reps. <30 seconds rest between sets and 60 seconds rest between exercises.

Choose a weight that is 40-65% of your one rep max weight with proper form.

Fat Burning Finishing Exercise:

Ski Jump-perform 4 sets of 25 reps

Set 1_____, Set 2 _____, Set 3_____, Set 4_____

Chapter 11

Putting It All Together

In the previous chapters I discussed numerous aspects to taking control of your male health, but where does one begin? In this chapter I will lay out step by step what you need to follow if you believe you may be suffering from low testosterone and what you can share with your physician to help you achieve an accurate diagnosis and more importantly the right therapy for you. Let's begin.

Step One: Take The Quiz

Taking inventory of your symptoms is a great place to start to understand what your body may be telling you.

Adam Questionnaire
Androgen Deficiency in the Aging Male (ADAM) Questionnaire

1. Do you have a decrease in sex drive?
2. Do you have a lack of energy?
3. Do you have a decrease in strength and/or endurance?
4. Have you lost height?
5. Have you noticed a decreased enjoyment in life?
6. Are you sad and/or grumpy?
7. Are your erections not as strong?
8. Has it been more difficult to maintain your erection throughout sexual intercourse?
9. Are you falling asleep after dinner?
10. Has your work performance deteriorated recently?

If you answered yes to number 1 or 7 or if you answer yes to more than 3 questions, you may have low testosterone. The next steps would be to make an appointment with your physician, share the questionnaire with him, and then get the labs so you can begin to evaluate your personal course of action.

Step Two: Go To The Doctor And Get Your Physical

Crucial to the process of getting the correct diagnosis, you need to have a face-to-face consultation with your physician which includes a physical exam. During this consultation your doctor should take note of your questionnaire and perform a thorough physical examination, which includes a testicular examination and a digital rectal examination of the prostate. I know no one really wants to have it done, however it is an important part of the physical exam and prostate cancer is the fifth leading cause of cancer death in men. Prostate cancer occurs in a little over 1 million men per year with an estimated number of deaths just over 300,000 per year. The prostate exam procedure is quick, painless, and you're done.

You may also want to share with your physician the nutritional questionnaires from chapter 8. These questionnaires offer a window into your body's current state of functioning and how well you may or may not be treating the only home you will ever really know - your own uniquely divine body. These questionnaires will help you gain insight into the degree of stress in your life and if you may be heading down the pathway to adrenal fatigue and dysfunction. You will also discover your personal allostatic load, which is the "wear and tear on the body" that heightens over time when you are exposed to repeated chronic stress, whether it is physical or emotional.

Stress hormones such as cortisol and epinephrine are the main hormonal mediators in the stress response and they can have both protective and damaging effects upon your body. When they are functioning appropriately they are essential for survival, however, if they are in constant demand due to ever-present chronic stress they can negatively affect the neuroendocrine system, immune system, digestive system, cardiovascular system, and central nervous system, disrupting your body's natural homeostasis.

The questionnaires will help you learn about your current state of digestion. This is critical to the absorption of nutrients, the status of your immune system, if your thyroid is functioning appropriately, if you consuming enough healthy fat, if your vitamin D levels up to par, if your sex hormones are in balance, and more.

Step Three: Get The Labs

So you've taken the quiz and answered yes to 3 or more of the questions indicating you may have low testosterone. Your body has been talking to you and you notice that you have low energy and don't have the get up and go to use to have, your libido has taken a vacation and that your erections are not as strong. You may also see you are gaining fat around the middle, your muscles are shrinking, and you're feeling like a grumpy old man. Your doctor has performed the physical exam and now it's time to get the right labs to make the diagnosis. When you have your laboratory performed what we're doing is gathering your personal biomarkers, which allows us to understand your current state of health. This health baseline will help not only to make the diagnosis but also to guide your therapy. I personally love looking at biomarkers as we are getting an intimate view of what is occurring inside your body. This information is invaluable, providing much more accuracy for a proper diagnosis. The following table below is the initial screening labs that should be ordered.

Initial Screening Labs:

- Total Testosterone
- Testosterone - Bioavailable or Weakly Bound
- Testosterone Free
- Cortisol AM
- SHBG
- HgA1c
- Thyroid Panel (TSH, FT4, FT3, rT3)
- LH/FSH
- DHT
- DHEA-Sulfate
- Sensitive Estradiol
- Liver panel
- Serum Chemistries
- CBC
- Lyme titer if relevant by history
- Insulin Immunoassay
- Lipid Panel or Lipoprotein panel
- Prolactin
- Vitamin D
- Cardiac CRP
- Homocysteine
- Iron
- TIBC
- Ferritin
- IGF-1
- IGF-BP3
- PSA
- Uric Acid
- Urinalysis

Biomarkers to Strongly Consider:

- IgG Food Sensitivity Testing
- Micronutrient Testing
- Lp-PLA2
- MPO
- NMR lipid, VAP, Berkley Heart Lab, or Cleveland Heart Lab
- MTHFR
- APOE

If you have a family history of an inherited blood clotting disorder or are not sure then you should consider these labs as well:

- Factor V Leiden mutation
- Factor VIII
- Factor XI
- Factor II (Prothrombin Gene)
- Fibrinogen
- Homocysteine

Labs to consider after initiation or follow up of testosterone replacement therapy:

These follow-up labs should be run at 3-4 weeks after starting therapy, changing therapy, or the delivery method. The same labs should also be performed at 3-month intervals during the first year and after the first year every 6 months or as necessary to monitor for unwanted side effects.

- Total Testosterone
- Sensitive Estradiol
- SHBG
- DHEA-S
- DHT
- FSH/LH
- Hemoglobin and Hematocrit
- Comprehensive Metabolic Panel
- PSA
- Bioavailable Testosterone or "Free and Loosely Bound"
- Free Testosterone if Bioavailable T is unavailable

Step Four: Understanding Some Of Your Labs

In my opinion this is the difficult part. Even after 19 years of providing testosterone replacement therapy and literally looking at thousands of lab results no two men are ever alike. The variations of lab results are seemingly endless and all their individual health goals are different, which is one reason as to why there will never be an acceptable "cookbook methodology" to the delivery of hormone replacement or for truly personalized care. This is why working with a skilled, experienced physician in testosterone replacement therapy who can deliver individualized personalized health care will pay off tenfold.

Now on to understanding some of the crucial labs, since the majority of individuals will be having serum blood levels tested I will discuss the following tests from that perspective.

Sex Hormone Binding Globulin

Sex hormone binding globulin, or SHBG, does exactly what it says - it binds sex hormones. Without knowing your sex hormone binding globulin level you cannot understand the levels of your sex hormones. Elevated SHBG issues can be somewhat more problematic and challenging causes of low bio available testosterone. Your SHBG is produced by the liver and bind both male and female hormones. Once these hormones are bound to sex hormone binding globulin they are unavailable for use because now they cannot bind to their appropriate hormone receptor.

So, higher sex hormone binding globulin lowers the bio available testosterone. The lower the sex hormone binding globulin level the greater the amount of free testosterone. Interestingly there is an order to which sex hormone binding globulin binds.

SHBG binds DHT > Testosterone > Androstenediol > Estradiol > Estrone

This demonstrates that sex hormone binding globulin has an affinity for the more androgenic hormones first. This means is that if both testosterone and estrogen are at equivalent levels, sex hormone binding globulin will bind more testosterone then estrogen making the level of bio available estrogen higher.

Unfortunately as we age the sex hormone binding globulin level and estrogen levels increase, while free testosterone levels and total testosterone levels decline. There is no real way to manipulate sex hormone binding globulin levels, though I have had some success with using Nettle Root 300 mg 3 times daily.

Factors that lower SHBG:

- Testosterone
- Growth hormone
- Prolactin
- Insulin
- Transcortin

Total Testosterone

Total testosterone is a fairly simple test that tells us the total testosterone concentration in the bloodstream at a given time. Ideally you like to have this lab drawn between 8 AM and 10 AM as the concentration of total testosterone will be at its highest. However this is just an isolated level of the total testosterone. Serum testosterone levels change throughout the day, and there is actually quite a bit of variability in the serum testosterone levels especially in younger men; but as we age that variability starts to decline. Variability of testosterone levels is actually a sign of good health. I like to see this level between 800-1200 pg/dL

A total testosterone less than 350 ng/dL is considered low, however symptoms can be felt at higher total testosterone levels. It is important to note that it is not the exact number but rather your clinical symptoms correlated with your numbers.

Now here is where sex hormone binding globulin comes into play. High levels of sex hormone binding globulin will bind testosterone making your free testosterone low and unavailable for use by the tissues. You can have a normal total testosterone level with high sex hormone binding globulin levels that then make free testosterone levels low and you suffer from the symptoms of low testosterone. While total testosterone is important for making dosage adjustments, it does not give us the complete clinical picture.

Bioavailable Testosterone

This is the actual amount of testosterone that is available for use in the body that can bind to the androgen receptors and cause the positive effects of this powerful hormone. Bioavailable testosterone is the sum of the free testosterone plus the loosely bound to albumin testosterone. Normal range for bio available testosterone is 40-250 ng/dL.

Free Testosterone

This is a measure of testosterone that is available to be used by the body. Free testosterone represents the actual amount of testosterone in the blood stream and ready to bind to receptor sites. I generally follow this value and like to see it in the range of 150-200 pg/dL

Androgen Metabolism

Testosterone is made in the testis and the adrenal glands. 5α-DHT is the most potent androgen, about three times more than testosterone, but it is primarily made within the liver and target cells and not by the testes. 5α-DHT is deactivated to 5α-androstanediol within target tissues and then conjugated for excretion. The corresponding beta metabolites, 5β-DHT and 5β- androstanediol are substantially less androgenic.

5α-Reductase Activity

The two enzymes 5α and 5β-reductase act on the androgen androstenedione which creates androsterone and etiocholanolone and testosterone that creates 5α-DHT and 5β-DHT. They also metabolize progesterone and cortisol. The alpha metabolites of androstenedione and testosterone are far more androgenic than their beta counterparts. An individual with increased 5α-reductase activity may have issues with excess facial hair growth, alopecia or hair loss, acne, oily skin and potential prostate issues.

Dihydrotestosterone-DHT/Prostate Specific Antigen-PSA

DHT or dihydrotestosterone is one of the breakdown products of testosterone caused by the 5 alpha reductase enzyme reactions. DHT further breaks down into 2 metabolites: 5β-DHT, which is the less androgenic form, and 5α-DHT, which is the more androgenic form responsible for oily skin, acne, prostate issues and male pattern baldness. If you happen to be a man who makes more 5α-DHT, saw palmetto can help reduce this more potent androgen. If you happen to be a man who makes more 5α-DHT and 4 hydroxyestrone, the genotoxic estrogen, this may possibly have negative prostate implications.

It is vitally important to measure DHT levels because higher levels of DHT can elevate your PSA. This level generally remains below 4 ng/mL. However, if the PSA starts to rise it is usually do to infection of the prostate or benign prostatic hyperplasia, which is an enlarged prostate or potentially prostate cancer.

It is advisable to have a baseline PSA and digital rectal examination at initiation of testosterone replacement therapy and then to repeat the PSA lab at 3 months after initiation of therapy and annually thereafter. If there are changes to the digital rectal exam or if there is a rise of greater than 0.35 ng/mL per year of the PSA velocity then a urologic consultation would be appropriate. If you are a man over 60 years of age with a rise of greater than 0.75 ng/mL per year of the PSA velocity, this would be an indication for urologic referral.

Estrogen

The other breakdown product of testosterone is estradiol or E2, which is a type of estrogen. As men age there is an increase in the conversion of testosterone to estrogen by the enzyme aromatase. The increase in estrogen many times leads to a simultaneous increase in SHBG, exacerbating the issue by binding more of the testosterone making it unavailable. What further complicates the issue is as men gain weight around their mid-section and fat accumulates their levels of aromatase increase causing further conversion of testosterone to estrogen.

Now estrogen has both "beneficial" and "unwanted" side effects on the alpha and beta-receptors within the cell affecting health, growth, and function of estrogen responsive tissues in the breasts, testes, prostate, brain, and bone.

Estrogen Metabolism

In regards to estrogen in men the primary concern is if they are making too much and which hydroxylation pathway their body prefers. Estrogens in men are produced from testosterone and androstenedione via aromatase activity.

The majority of estrogen is hydroxylated down a protective pathway creating 2-hydroxyestrone (2-OH-E1). This estrogen metabolite is considered protective in both women and men and is the preferred pathway leading to methylation and subsequent excretion of metabolites. However, phase 1 hydroxylation can take two other pathways: one towards 16-hydroxyestrone (16-OH-E1), the bad, or 4-hydroxyestrone (4-OH-E1), the ugly. Neither of these estrogen metabolites is desirable, with 16-OH-E1 exerting negative effects on the alpha and beta receptors triggering expression of target genes within the cell affecting the growth and function of estrogen responsive tissue in the prostate, breast, and testes. 4-OH-E1 is considered carcinogenic and its methylation to 4-methyoxyestrone (4-MeO) leading to excretion is the most desirable protective pathway for this potentially genotoxic metabolite.

In the example on the next page you can see that this man makes a large amount of the beneficial 2-OH-E1 (bottom of the report, center), but also makes a large amount of 4-OH-E1 (left of the 2nd pie chart) as well. Fortunately he has strong methylation activity (bottom center left), however some nutrition adjustment and judicious use of aromatase inhibitors can improve his profile even further. Remember chapter 7, heal your gut and detox your liver? This is why healthy liver function of phase 1 hydroxylation and phase 2 methylation is so important in the clearing of estrogen and its metabolites.

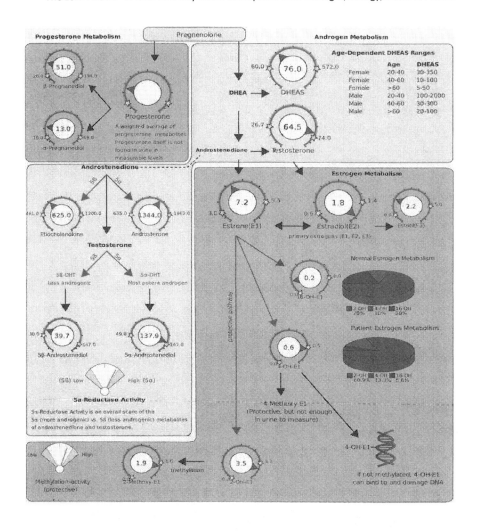

By now you have probably noticed that the lab I like to follow is the sensitive estradiol. This is an important point because the standard estradiol test will overestimate the amount of estrogen in the man's system, leading to possible inappropriate aromatase inhibitor usage. Over the years I have performed both standard and sensitive estradiol tests on clients and the results are always different. Below is a patient's standard and sensitive estradiol assays and at the time he was having headaches and some joint aches, both symptoms of low estrogen. Stopping the aromatase inhibitor did the trick.

Estradiol   View Official Report

Estradiol	27.6	pg/mL	7.6-42.6
	Roche ECLIA methodology		

Estradiol, Sensitive   View Official Report

Estradiol, Sensitive	9	pg/mL	3-70

Male Female 0- 6 yrs. 0 - 15 0 - 15 7-10 yrs. 0 - 15 0 - 70 11-12 yrs. 0 - 40 10 - 300 13-15 yrs. 0 - 45 10 - 300 >15 yrs. 3 - 70 See Below Ovulating Female Follicular Phase 9 - 175 Luteal Phase 44 - 196 Periovulatory 107 - 281 Oral Contraceptives 0 - 91 Postmenopausal Treated 42 - 289 Untreated 0 - 19 . Estradiol results obtained with different assay methods cannot be used interchangeably. It is recommended that only one assay method be used consistently to monitor serial patient results.

Prolactin

Prolactin is a hormone release from the pituitary gland and when prolactin is too high it can cause hypogonadism. The most common cause being a pituitary tumor that is called an adenoma and it is not cancerous but it is a cause of low testosterone. Such things as eating and having sex can also elevate prolactin. There are also common medications, which can elevate prolactin such as antidepressants, opioids, calcium channel blockers, and other medications.

Luteinizing Hormone-LH

Luteinizing hormone is produced by the pituitary gland and makes way to the testicles where it stimulates the Leydig cells to produce testosterone. If the hypothalamic-pituitary-testicular axis is intact and LH levels surge, more testosterone is produced when LH levels decrease less testosterone is produced. The release of luteinizing hormone is pulsatile in nature and as we age frequency and strength of the pulsatile release decreases contributing to andropause.

The initial picture we usually see in the late 30s and early 40s is one of hypogonadotropic hypogonadism. This is a low GnRH (gonadotropic releasing hormone) released from the hypothalamus with a low LH released from the pituitary and low testosterone released from the testicles. This is where natural therapies such as lifestyle modification, exercise, and strategic supplementation can optimize the natural production of testosterone, delaying the need for direct hormone replacement and where HCG therapy is a most valuable player. Inevitably at some future date the system will start to fail and that is when we have an andropause, or what the media likes to call "manopause". The clinical picture generally now is one of low testosterone with high LH and high

GnRH or hypergonadotropic hypogonadism, which means you are on the downhill slope to no longer feeling like the man you used to be. Sometimes the changes are rapid and noticeable and other times the changes are so slow you do not notice until one day you wake up looking in the mirror wondering when the former you disappeared.

Follicle Stimulating Hormone-FSH

Follicle-stimulating hormone is another gonadotropic hormone that is less pulsatile than LH and has a longer half-life. FSH can be valuable in evaluating the hypothalamic pituitary testicular axis.

DHEA-S

In the blood we monitor DHEA-S. DHEA is an important player in the overall health and wellness of both men and women with strong benefits related to neurocognitive function, cardiovascular health, sex drive, muscle development, and immune health. DHEA is metabolized into both estrogen and testosterone and adding it to the treatment regime should not be taken lightly as the downstream metabolites could cause issues if dosed incorrectly and not monitored. There are multiple delivery methods that include gels, creams, capsule, sublingual spray, and troche.

CBC/Chemistries

At the initial evaluation and all follow ups a CBC is necessary for baseline evaluation of the hemoglobin and hematocrit. One of the potential side effects of testosterone replacement therapy in particular injectable testosterone is that it can stimulate bone marrow production of red blood cells by enhancing production of erythropoietin stimulating factor. In approximately 5-7% of patients this increased production is enough to cause erythrocytosis (increased red blood cells), necessitating the cessation of testosterone replacement therapy or therapeutic phlebotomy. If your hemoglobin exceeds 18.0 and hematocrit exceeds 55.0 then therapy needs to be withheld and or blood donation considered.

At the initial evaluation serum chemistries should be drawn as well to identify any abnormalities and to have a baseline to refer as necessary. In my experience it is not unusual to discover abnormalities in the serum chemistries such as having a low magnesium level that contribute to low testosterone.

Homocystiene

Many of you have probably never heard of this amino acid injury and are wondering what this has to do with low testosterone. High homocystiene levels are a marker for inflammation. This nasty little amino acid damages the endothelial lining of the artery and contributes significantly the incidence of heart disease, stroke and Alzheimer's disease. If your body has difficulty absorbing B vitamins or you have a lifestyle with poor diet and excessive alcohol that contributes to decreased absorption of nutrients, then high levels of homocystiene are contributing to your disease burden. Remember if the blood doesn't flow the sex is a no go!

HgbA1c

HgbA1c levels indicate how well your blood sugars have been controlled over the last 3-4 months. Imagine for a minute that your red blood cells are like a doughnut. Healthy red blood cells are like a plain doughnut; however unhealthy red blood cells are like a doughnut with sprinkles. High levels indicate risk for the development of diabetes. Numerous studies have demonstrated the serious effects of consistently elevated HgbA1c levels on the oxidation of LDL cholesterol. Epidemiologic studies have shown that higher levels are associated with substantially higher risks for congestive heart failure, heart disease, heart attacks, strokes, brain atrophy, cancer, vascular endothelial dysfunction, increased blood clotting, high blood pressure, diabetes, and thyroid disorders. It is strongly recommended to identify and treat impaired fasting glucose early as its progression into diabetes and coronary artery disease is silent and progressive until a catastrophic event occurs. Ideally you want a hemoglobin A1c level of 5 percent or lower.

Cardiac CRP Or HS-CRP

Cardiac CRP or high sensitivity CRP which stands for C-reactive protein is a direct measure of inflammation of the endothelial lining inside the blood vessels. Increased inflammation of the endothelial lining attributes to the buildup of plaque and increases your risk of heart attack or stroke. Back to that blood flow again!

Iron/Tibc/Ferritin

At the initial evaluation it is essential to screen for excessive iron, total iron binding capacity, and elevated ferritin levels which can contribute to low testosterone.

Hemochromatosis, which is an inherited disease that causes an enhanced gastrointestinal absorption of iron, leads to iron accumulation in numerous organs to include the skin, joints, pancreas, heart and the testicles, which can cause hypogonadism and low testosterone. Also non-intentional excessive iron intake whether it is from supplements or from a contaminated water supply can also lead to decreased testosterone production.

Liver Panel

The liver is a vitally important organ where glucose is converted into energy. The liver also manages the storage of glucose in muscle and plays a role in the creation of fat. One of the main jobs is to process or detox whatever you eat or drink, medications or supplements that you take, or toxins that enter your body. The liver function tests are AST, ALT and GGT.

Vitamin D

Vitamin D is present in numerous cells throughout the body and plays a role in the immune system, brain function, mood stability, bone health and cardiovascular health. It is one of the most common nutritional deficiencies that I see on a daily basis. Excessive alcohol consumption, not enough time spent outdoors or poor nutrition habits all lead to this deficiency. If vitamin D were exclusive to one pharmaceutical company, I would be their biggest prescriber! Here in Midwest Ohio everyone is deficient. In general I like my patients to have vitamin D levels that reach 60-80 international units. Generally, I use vitamin D3 ranging from 1000 international units - 10,000 international units per day depending on the patient and their individual needs. If you have trouble absorbing vitamin D3 a prescription for vitamin D2 (ergocalciferol) may be in order. If you suffer from a mood disorder correcting a vitamin D deficiency may be beneficial, I have personally seen numerous individuals' lives change drastically with simple vitamin D supplementation.

Lyme Titer

If you are an outdoorsman and you have a history of a tick bite, I highly recommend having a Lyme titer. Lyme disease is due to a spirochete, borrelia burgdorferi and is a disease resulting in body wide inflammation. I have seen several cases of undiagnosed Lyme disease presented to my office with complaints of low testosterone. The most dramatic was a man with a Bell's palsy (facial drooping on one side) who came into the office complaining of low testosterone only to discover he had Lyme disease he contracted during a fishing trip in upper New York State.

Factor V Leiden Mutation/Factor Viii/Factor Xi/Fibrinogen

If you have a family history of an inherited blood clotting disorder, a personal history of blood clots or are not sure then you should consider these labs as well:

The Dynamic Dou: Adrenal & Thyroid Function

Free T3 & T4, TSH

The thyroid gland is responsible for how quickly the body uses energy and makes proteins. The two hormones that it makes are free T3 and free T4 and they are responsible for regulating metabolism as well as the rate of function of other systems in the body. TSH or thyroid-stimulating hormone, which is released from the anterior pituitary, stimulates the thyroid gland to release free T3 and free T4. Measuring all 3 hormones is necessary to evaluate the functioning of the thyroid gland.

Cortisol

Cortisol is a hormone secreted by the adrenal glands released under emotional or physical stress that directly affects your blood sugar. When your body is under stress, either physical or psychological, your HPA-axis (hypothalamic-pituitary-adrenal axis) is encouraged to produce ACTH (adrenocorticotropic hormone) which stimulates the adrenal glands to make the stress hormone cortisol and to a some extent DHEA-S. The majority of cortisol is then metabolized to "metabolized cortisol". One needs to examine the levels of both "free" and "metabolized" cortisol to correctly assess adrenal function.

In healthy adrenal function, the daily free cortisol levels are expected to rise in the morning and fall throughout the day, reaching the lowest point right after going to sleep.

Any event that raises your cortisol to high levels can have detrimental effects upon your blood sugar metabolism, which causes you to store energy as fat. This is one piece of the puzzle as to why you get fat deposits around your midsection as you age.

Step Five: Consider These Powerful Diagnostic Tests

Vo2 Assessment

A VO2 Max test involves a graded exercise test on a treadmill or on a bike. The test begins at a very light intensity and gets slightly harder each minute until maximum exertion. The subject wears a mask and we measure the volume of air expired along with the percentages of oxygen and carbon dioxide in the expired air. From this data, we can determine the following:

Aerobic Threshold:

Aerobic threshold is the optimal intensity (wattage, running speed and/or heart-rate) for developing endurance. At aerobic threshold intensity, the body is recruiting almost all of the slow-twitch muscle fibers, but not yet recruiting any of the fast twitch fibers. Most individuals, without the benefit of physiological testing, overestimate this intensity. Using optimal intensity for basic endurance training maximizes fat burning and minimizes recovery time and injury risk. Most individuals perform basic endurance workouts at an intensity that is too high. Conducting basic endurance workouts at optimal intensity is much more efficient, enabling increased training volume as well as greater frequency and better quality workouts.

Lactate Threshold:

Known as the red-line to endurance athletes, this threshold is the highest intensity at which the body can recycle lactic acid as quickly as it is produced. Just below lactate threshold (LT), an athlete is working hard and acid levels are moderately high, but it does not accumulate. Speeding up just a little will cause lactic acid accumulation. Knowing this precise threshold enables an individual to work out most efficiently.

Lactic acid is a byproduct of exercise, which makes the muscles burn, and may contribute to fatigue. During exercise, even at low intensity, we are always producing lactic acid. Individuals' muscles are also constantly burning lactic acid and using it as a fuel. At low intensity the muscles easily recycle as much acid as is produced. The higher the intensity is, the more acid the muscles produce. At lactate threshold intensity, the muscle is able to recycle the acid as quickly as it is produced. If the individual speeds up just slightly, the muscles produce more acid than it can recycle and acid accumulates, causing fatigue and damaging the muscles.
VO2 Max:

VO2 Max is the volume of oxygen the body uses during one minute of maximal exercise. This data tells your potential for endurance. While aerobic and lactate thresholds are the best predictors of current endurance performance, VO2 Max is one indicator of an individual's potential.

Carotid Ultrasound & Carotid Intima-Media Thickness (CIMT)

CIMT is a noninvasive ultrasound test that is being recommended by the American Heart Association and the American College of Cardiology to screen for heart disease in apparently healthy individuals ages 45 or greater. The carotid arteries provide a "window" to the coronary arteries. Not only do they have similar risk factors - more importantly, the relationship between the atherosclerotic burden in a carotid artery and a coronary artery is the same as between any two coronary arteries. Therefore carotid atherosclerosis provides a window into the amount of coronary atherosclerosis in an individual. CIMT is an independent predictor of future cardiovascular events, including heart attacks, cardiac death, and stroke.

Neurocognitive Assessment

Neurocognitive testing is a method clinicians use to assess a patient's memory, mental speed and other cognitive functions. Individuals with hormone deficiencies, elevated inflammatory markers, and genetic mutations such as MTHFR are at greater risk for dementia and neurocognitive assessment gives us an ability to detect early decline.

DEXA Scan

DEXA stands for dual energy X-Ray absorptiometry. It is a totally safe, painless, noninvasive way to measure bone density and determine total body fat. The amount of x-ray exposure from DEXA is less than 1/10th of the dose you would get from an ordinary chest x-ray. Men and women with endocrine disorders, such as low growth hormone, low testosterone, high thyroid hormone (Grave's Disease), high cortisol hormone (Cushing's Syndrome), and hyperparathyroidism can also experience bone loss leading to osteoporosis.

Osteoporosis can lead to hip fractures and spontaneous vertebral fractures, which lead to loss of height. Both of these are easily prevented if the diagnosis is made early. There are various therapies available to treat osteoporosis. The earlier that therapy is initiated the less likely the patient is to develop fractures.

Arterial Occlusion Testing

Arterial occlusion testing is a noninvasive diagnostic device used to measure vascular reactivity for early detection of cardiovascular disease and monitoring response to therapy. The test begins with an automated blood pressure measurement, followed by cuff occlusion of the right arm. During the cuff occlusion (2 to 5 minutes), fingertip temperature in the right hand falls because of the absence of warm circulating blood. Once the cuff is released, blood flow rushes into the forearm and hand, causing a temperature rebound in the fingertip, which is directly proportional to the vascular reactivity. Vascular dysfunction is considered to be the earliest clinically detectable stage of subclinical atherosclerosis.

Step Six: The Natural Options

If you're a man in your 30s and 40s and your laboratory panel discloses a hypogonadotropic hypogonadism, in other words a low GnRH, low LH, and low testosterone then natural therapies such as lifestyle modification, exercise, strategic nutrition and supplementation can optimize the natural production of testosterone delaying the need for direct hormone replacement. This approach can help your body's natural ability to maintain hormonal homeostasis for an indefinite period of time until the time arrives that you enter andropause. The hypothalamic-pituitary-testicular axis has an amazing ability to regain its plasticity if nurtured in the correct environment.

This is where you should begin. The hypothalamic-pituitary-testicular axis is an amazing, delicate and intricate dance of multiple hormones and you should take every step possible to maintain this balance until the very end when it becomes necessary to exert outside control. As a man and as a physician skilled in the arts and science of hormone replacement my preference always is and always will be to attempt to maintain this delicate balance. It is helpful to be strategic and this is where intracellular nutrient testing, food sensitivity testing and advanced hormone tests can make a monumental difference. *Refer to chapter five for the necessary steps to take to regain control.*

I know you are wondering, "Why can't you just tell me what to take?" Good question and that is because there is no cookbook for this approach. Every man is different and every man we see at the Alpha Male Medical Institute is built a personalized plan to help him reach his natural hormonal best. No two men ever present with the same intracellular nutrient deficiencies, food sensitivities, preexisting disease states and severity of disease, mental status, hormone status, or functional status of their multiple axes.

Each man is unto himself a unique composite of his current time and place in his personal health continuum, which requires a personalized, precise, and ever adapting approach to achieve constant health and vitality.

Step Seven: The HCG Option – Human Chorionic Gonadotropin

When purely natural options fail to regain control of your testosterone levels, under the correct circumstance HCG is a powerful stimulator of the testicles to help them manufacture testosterone. The administration of HCG will stimulate the production of endogenous testosterone. This is because the alpha subunit of HCG and luteinizing hormone are identical, which means that it acts as an LH analog. An additional benefit of the use of HCG is that it preserves testicular size and sperm count. HCG is a purified natural hormone from the urine of pregnant women. HCG is simple to use with a low side effect profile and often amazing results. A simple injection into the abdomen with a small insulin needle twice each week is all you need. Dosages can range anywhere from 500 international units to 5000 international units twice each week.

Your physician needs to follow your laboratory 4 weeks after initiation of therapy and at intervals of 3 months. You and your physician should discuss your results along with how you are feeling overall because what is important is not what the lab values show but how you are responding and feeling with treatment. The overall goal is to achieve hormonal balance and enhance your vitality and health. Combined HCG therapy along with healthful nutrition, stimulating exercise, appropriate supplementation and hydration, adequate rest and the increase in testosterone will go to work producing lean muscle and a healthier functioning metabolism. HCG is a great way to enhance the production of testosterone until the testicles stop responding to this analog hormone. What happens at this point is that testosterone levels begin to decline again and the man slides into andropause. This is when I usually change men over to testosterone or combination therapy.

Step Eight: Testosterone Replacement Therapy

My step wise approach to improving a man's level of testosterone starts with natural therapies that involve the use of specific nutritional plans, strategic personalized supplementation, meaningful exercise, sleep hygiene and advanced testing. When this approach is either on a downslope or failing, I make the move to HCG or testosterone. If HCG was my first choice, I will continue with HCG until it no longer can deliver which at that time I then add testosterone to the treatment regime.

Testosterone has several potential delivery methods and any doctor can make any of these modalities work. All are completely acceptable delivery methods but they all have their own technical advantages and disadvantages, however my personal preference is that of injection. It is simple; it can be done at home, it is reliable, consistent, predictable, and it is easy to measure.

Listed below are the many delivery options for testosterone replacement therapy. I have placed them in the order from my lowest preference to highest.

The Subcutaneous Implant

Small pellets no larger than a grain of rice are implanted under the skin through a small incision in either the buttocks or the abdomen. I implanted pellets for a few years and after monitoring hundreds of lab values and patients and the numerous side effects and complications, I ceased this procedure. In my opinion pellet therapy is barbaric and far from physiologic. It results in huge variations in testosterone levels that are not in balance with the body. There is no way to make appropriate adjustments to therapy at any given time; you have to wait 3-6 months for pellet degradation. Over the years I have seen numerous unwanted side effects from pellet therapy to include; supraphysiologic testosterone levels, anxiety, extreme agitation, expulsion of pellets, infection, adrenal exhaustion, scarring, fibrosis, ilioinguinal neuropathy and more. I realize there are those physicians and patients that prefer this method, but they are no longer used for my clients or myself and I recommend you not use them either.

Buccal Patch

A small tablet is placed between the cheek and gum a couple times a day to deliver the testosterone; the benefit is that it is supposed to avoid entering the stomach and potential liver toxicity. I would not recommend this method.

Transdermal Patch

A skin patch that is coated with medicine that can be applied to the scrotum or upper arm, which supplies a steady stream of testosterone to the patient. Inevitably the patch causes skin irritation not to mention usually high levels of DHT, which can lead to unwanted complications. I would not recommend this method.

Topical Gel and Cream

These transdermal delivery systems are available in pumps, packets, Topi-CLICK® measured-dose applicators and other delivery systems. The gel and cream can be applied to the upper arms and shoulders or to the inner forearms, which are then rubbed against the sides of the body, which is the method I teach to my patients. It is best to allow time for the gel or cream to dry on the skin completely. You can either do once or twice daily dosing and both preparations create a nice variability in serum androgen levels. Some will argue that gel is better than cream however I have had excellent results with both preparations, so it is a matter of preference. Care needs to be taken not to accidently transfer to women and children. The downside to these preparations is that they can lead to higher levels of both estrogen and DHT because their respective converting enzymes reside in high concentration in the skin. This can be problematic for those who make larger concentrations of either 5α-DHT or 4-OH-E1 or 16-OH-E1 and who have poor methylation activity. For the needle phobic individual these are definitely the way to go and I highly recommend them as a delivery system.

Intramuscular or Subcutaneous Injection

Delivery of testosterone via either intramuscular or subcutaneous injection is my preferred route of administration. Injection of testosterone into either the upper outer quadrant of the buttock can be subcutaneous or intramuscular depending on the individual. One could also use the lower anterior abdomen for subcutaneous administration or injection into the upper outer vastus lateralis muscle in the thigh for intramuscular injection; both are simply accomplished with minimal discomfort. There is nice variability in testosterone levels from day to day which mimics the body's natural state and serum blood levels are easily followed.

In general I use testosterone cypionate suspended in either cottonseed oil or grape seed oil and occasionally utilize testosterone enanthate suspended in sesame oil for those individuals that have sensitivities to testosterone cypionate.

I educate my patients on self-injection techniques to eliminate the need for frequent office visits, as this is substantially more convenient, especially if the patient is on a micro dose schedule of injections. I utilize a one-piece tuberculin syringe with a 25 gauge 5/8-inch needle for subcutaneous injection or a 25 gauge 1 inch for intramuscular injections.

The benefits of injection therapy are significant. Ease of administration, low cost, can do at home, produces reliable blood levels, dosage amounts and dosing regimen can be easily adjusted, can mimic natural variability, low side effect profile that is predictable, predictable onset of action and time course to benefits, and the list goes on which makes testosterone delivered by injection whether subcutaneous or intramuscular the winner in my book.

Whichever therapy you chose to utilize you must be monitored by your physician for potential side effects from therapy. Upon initiation of therapy or changes in dosing regimen at 4 weeks and then every 3 months thereafter for the first year of therapy. After the first year of therapy the monitoring interval can be broadened at the discretion of the physician.

The most common unwanted side effects from testosterone therapy:

- Testicular shrinkage
- Decrease in HDL (good) cholesterol
- Polycythemia or increased red blood cells
- Gynecomastia or Breast enlargement
- Decrease in sperm count
- Acne
- Worsening sleep Apnea
- Edema (swelling)

Your physician can easily address all of these potential side effects. Now after many years of delivering testosterone to hypogonadal men the most common side effect to be addressed in my experience is testicular shrinkage, which is easily managed with HCG. There is potential for a nominal decrease in HDL, I have never seen any dramatic decrease. Polycythemia occurs in about 5% of men and is easily managed by stopping therapy, adjusting therapy, or blood donation. Decrease in sperm count for the majority of men is a non-issue, if the desire for pregnancy arises, switching to HCG can help. I have NEVER seen a case of gynecomastia caused by appropriate testosterone replacement therapy; I have however seen dozens of individuals with gynecomastia caused by the illegal use of steroids in multiple forms by young men, and quite dramatic.

Potential Medication Interactions:

Beta Blockers: testosterone therapy often increases clearance of the medication requiring an increase in dosage

Oxyphenbutazone: testosterone therapy decreases the clearance of the medication requiring lowering of the dosage

Medications for Diabetes: testosterone therapy often times decreases the amount of medication needed.

Contraindications to Testosterone Replacement Therapy

- Cancer of the Breast
- Cancer of the Prostate, which now may be only in specific patient cases
- Untreated Pituitary Tumors

It is important to remember that every man's body is different in numerous ways that go beyond the explanation of current science. That being said, what works well for one man may be completely ineffective for another man - which is why it is always best to take a personalized approach to your health and wellness. My dear friend and colleague Dr. Florence Comite, author of the bestselling book *"Keep It Up"* refers to this approach as precision medicine, and I could not agree more.

Step Nine: Dealing With Excess Estrogen

One of the potential issues in testosterone replacement therapy is excess estrogen. Elevated estrogen can lead to several issues such as:

- Nipple sensitivity
- Elevation of SHBG
- Decreased libido
- Infertility
- Mood Instability
- Vasospasm
- Increased Clotting
- Swelling
- Cancers-questionable
- Prostate swelling
- Accumulation of fat
- Breast growth

It is best to wait until after the 4 week follow up labs to evaluate how your body is metabolizing your testosterone therapy before the initiation of an aromatase inhibitor such as Arimidex. It is not possible to predict which way a man's body will preferentially metabolize the testosterone, and in many an instance I have seen a man's estrogen stay mid-range and in balance with therapy. Driving the estrogen too low can have detrimental effects as well such as headaches, mood instability, loss of libido, cardiovascular effects, changes in lipid metabolism, vascular endothelial effects, bone health, joint aches and pains.

Decreasing the dosage of testosterone or adjusting the dose of other hormones such as DHEA can also effectively reduce levels of estrogen. If an aromatase inhibitor is needed it is best to start low and slow as the saying goes.

Step Ten: Dealing With Excess DHT

Dihydrotestosterone (DHT), the other downstream by-product of testosterone metabolism must also be monitored closely as levels may increase with testosterone replacement therapy. DHT is a very potent androgen that drives libido. 5α-DHT is the more androgenic form responsible for oily skin, acne, benign prostatic hypertrophy, and male pattern baldness. If there are no adverse symptoms with a higher DHT level then it is generally recommend withholding therapy with a 5 alpha reductase inhibitor.

There are other safer approaches to lowering DHT levels, such as changing the delivery system from a gel or cream to injectable, or reduction of the dosage supplementation with saw palmetto. 5 alpha reductase inhibitors have the potential to quite negatively affect a man's libido so every caution should be made to avoid these unless absolutely necessary.

The Bad Hat Trick: Hypogonadism, Adrenal Dysfunction, And Low Functioning Thyroid

The hat trick in sports circles signifies 3 positive events in a row; unfortunately what I call the bad hat trick is something entirely different and a health state where you never want to find yourself. Over the past few years I have noticed a common thread of 3 glandular dysfunctions occurring in some men with severe fatigue, no sex drive, muscle wasting, weight loss and or weight gain, and overall poor health. More often than not the man has been diagnosed with low testosterone and has been treated in the past or is currently being treated for low testosterone with no perceived benefit.

Often I find that these individuals are suffering from low testosterone, low adrenal function, and a low functioning thyroid and the severity of their symptoms can be quite dramatic. These men are often very difficult to treat because of their overlapping low functioning adrenal glands, thyroid gland, and low testosterone.

It is crucial to understand the relationship between the adrenal glands and the thyroid gland. The adrenal gland relies on the thyroid gland to function adequately. Most every cell in your body has receptors for both thyroid and cortisol hormones. Cortisol is produced in the adrenal cortex and thyroid is produced in the thyroid gland. If you have low thyroid function you will have low adrenal function, which means a low production of cortisol and aldosterone. Which means you will often have difficulty with sodium and potassium retention, which can lead to weakness, fatigue, low blood pressure, weak pulse, dizziness, and even difficulty standing. Because you have low cortisol levels your thyroid will not function as well and the conversion of T4 to the active T3 will be decreased. Cortisol assists the thyroid gland in working more efficiently. Thyroid hormones are crucial for appropriate adrenal function and optimal cortisol levels. As you can see there is a critical relationship between your thyroid gland and your adrenal glands.

The thyroid gland, located at the base of the front of the neck, is the engine that drives metabolism in that it helps process food and energy. When your metabolism isn't working correctly everything in your body slows down, and that means that every gland, organ, and every cell is affected. As your thyroid function slows down so do your adrenal glands, creating stress in your body; thus causing an increase in your adrenaline output and further creating more stress on the adrenal glands. Low thyroid function also leads to an increase in cortisol binding globulin, which further binds cortisol making it unavailable for use to every cell in the body. Low thyroid function even slows down the detoxification process in the liver, which can prevent the breakdown products of cortisol and estrogen from being cleared from your body.

Cortisol is a glucocorticoid that affects the metabolism of carbohydrates, fats and protein. Cortisol promotes the breakdown of protein to amino acids, opposes insulin by inhibiting cellular glucose uptake and oxidation, decreases calcium levels, suppresses the immune system, promotes the breakdown of triacylglycerol in adipose tissue to glycerol and fatty acids, and supports the action of growth hormone and glucagon. Cortisol helps keep the body's reaction to stress in perfect balance and also has a function in increasing blood sugar levels by the breakdown of the macronutrients, proteins, carbohydrates, and fats to help make energy that reaches every cell in the body.

If you are man who has low testosterone, adrenal dysfunction, and low thyroid there is a specific order in which treatment must be started. I have observed that you must first heal the adrenal glands before healing the thyroid gland and treating the low testosterone. If you increase the metabolic rate from the addition of thyroid hormone and/or testosterone before healing the adrenal glands you will often make the adrenal dysfunction worse. It is best to recover the adrenal glands first then treat the low functioning thyroid and then the low testosterone.

Tips to heal the Adrenals

- No coffee or alcohol
- No nicotine
- No sugar
- No processed foods
- Drink plenty of water
- Strategic exercise that limits heart rate, best determined by VO2 testing, in general do not exceed a heart rate of 120 beats per minute during exercise for a period of 30-90 days depending on severity of symptoms

- Eat small frequent meals
- Bedtime 10:00-10:30
- Practice Sleep hygiene

Supplement with:

- Vitamin D3
- Vitamin C
- N-acetylcystiene
- Digestive enzymes (lipase, amylase, protease, pepsin, betaine)
- Vitamin B5 (pyridoxine)
- Vitamin B6 (pantothenic acid)
- Citrus bioflavonoids
- Warm water with sea salt
- Porcine or bovine glandular support
- Licorice

Tips to heal the Thyroid

- No coffee or alcohol
- No nicotine
- No sugar
- No processed foods
- Drink plenty of water
- Eat small frequent meals
- Bedtime 10:00-10:30
- Practice Sleep hygiene
- Sublingual Iodine drops under the guidance of a physician

Conclusion

In bringing this chapter and the book to a close I wanted to make commentary about the field of age management medicine, hormone therapy and lifestyle intervention. Before embarking on a journey that includes hormone replacement therapy it would be best to ensure that you have a complete and thorough history and physical, laboratory, and all necessary ancillary testing completed to gather as many biomarkers as possible for your physician before starting any kind of hormone replacement therapy.

In my opinion there is an overabundance of readily available "testosterone clinics" who will be more than happy to inappropriately place you on hormone therapy with only doing the bare minimum of testing to make a "lone diagnosis" of low testosterone for the sole purpose of revenue generation with no regard to the impact of unnecessary hormones on your overall health and wellness. This is not good medicine and hormones do not function in isolation. Quite the opposite is true, for every adjustment you make there will be a downstream reaction and effect to the addition or deletion of a hormone.

There are dozens of reasons that cause an individual to have low testosterone from environmental influences, viruses, chronic illness, heavy metal toxicity, tumors, excess binding hormones, poor nutrition habits, lifestyle habits, excessive exercise and many more. Choosing the path of not investigating the cause of the hormone deficiency or excess and merely moving straight ahead to treatment with the "biggest tool in the tool box", testosterone is not in your best interest. The unwanted side effects of inappropriate testosterone usage can have permanent lifelong implications.

Many times I am able to recover an individual's hypothalamic-pituitary-testicular-axis with strategic changes in nutrition, lifestyle, and supplementation to completely rebuild this intricate and delicate process. It is always best to keep the body in balance and let it do what it likes to do naturally. No human intervention can ever hope to replicate this incredibly complex dance of hormones that has been divinely orchestrated. It would be with great hubris to ever think that man could ever come close to replicating what nature does so well.

One only has to look to the world of bodybuilding to see such egotism and flagrant disregard for the miracle of human life and all its complexities. Steroid abuse abounds in every gym, community, and athletic event across our country and around the world. All the while quietly in the background many of the current and one time illegal steroid users suffer from numerous unwanted side effects such as tendon ruptures, infections, abscesses, Hepatitis B and C, liver tumors and cancer, gynecomastia, heart arrhythmias, derangement of cholesterol profiles leading to atherosclerosis, heart attacks, strokes and more.

If you are a young man contemplating the use of illegal steroids and you are reading this book, take heed. Over the years I have seen numerous men come through my doors having abused illegal steroids. These were some of the biggest, burliest men weeping like babies over the permanent side effects caused by their abuse. I have seen marriages destroyed and lives ruined by the inappropriate and illegal use of steroids. Be stronger than them. It takes a weak man to say yes to the temptation and a strong man to say no. Be a strong man and stay clean, eat healthy, exercise strategically, get adequate rest and use supplements wisely and sparingly. When the time comes as you age and andropause affects you and it becomes necessary to make the decision as to whether or not to pursue testosterone replacement therapy, it will deliver the medical results you need.

Early in my medical career I took a strong interest in the functioning of the brain, and part of that process is how the brain manufactures and releases hormones to communicate with every organ, tissue, and cell in the body. I was truly amazed that such small glands like the hypothalamus, the pituitary, thyroid, adrenals, ovaries, and testicles could exert such incredible control and function throughout the human body. Unfortunately, through medical school, internship, and residency very little education and time is spent discussing these intricate processes and what to do when things go wrong. We really had very little training in hormone physiology and our teaching physicians were not really familiar with the use of testosterone. So I took upon myself to learn everything I could that had to do with male health and wellness. It really seemed like a good fit, being athletically inclined and always being drawn to pushing my body as far as it would go, especially with triathlons.

For many years there has always been a negative light shown around testosterone replacement therapy because of an incorrect assumption that somehow testosterone caused prostate cancer. This assumption is incorrect and not true. We now know because of the work of many individuals that prostate cancer risk actually goes up as our testosterone levels fall as we age. We all have our heroes and some of mine include Dr. Eugene Shippen, author of *"The Testosterone Syndrome"*, Dr. Jeffry Life author of *"The Life Plan"* and *"Mastering the Life Plan"* and a physician by the name of Abraham Morgentaler, M.D. author of *"Testosterone for Life"*, who is a urologist in Boston that has spent his entire career researching the potential positive and negative effects of testosterone replacement therapy. He has published many articles related to testosterone replacement therapy and his body of research has found no evidence that men who have high testosterone levels are at risk or greater risk of prostate cancer. Actually, quite the opposite was found to be true, the lower your testosterone levels the greater your risk for prostate cancer as you age.

This brings me to important point. In medicine and in life you must always seek the truth for many an incorrect assumption made by singular study will often dictate care literally for decades until the truth finally comes out. In my mind you must always question "what was" and "what is". **Currently the question that I get asked is; "does testosterone cause heart attacks and strokes?"** This question is being asked because of all the media attention and dramatization around a couple of misguided, observational studies which in the opinion of many in the field of andrology see as non-informative. There are hundreds of studies that show the benefits of optimizing low hormones and not just testosterone. Taking a proactive approach to your health care, identifying your biomarkers that are in decline or excess, obtaining the appropriate ancillary testing, and then personalizing your program to meet your needs leads to having more energy, leaner and stronger muscles, a high functioning metabolism, and improved overall health and well-being. Your blood pressure will improve, your cholesterol profile will improve, your body's ability to metabolize sugar will improve, you will have more energy, you'll feel stronger, you'll feel more confident about who you and your sex drive will go through the roof!

There will never be a one-size fit all approach that will work in personalized health care. Achieving the best results in your health care means working in concert with your physician, monitoring your biomarkers, making changes in your lifestyle, nutrition, and exercise habits, optimizing your hormones and supplements and making the commitment to your personal program of superior health and fitness.

To Your Health And Vitality,

Dr. Rob Kominiarek

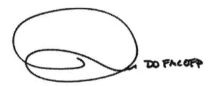

About The Author

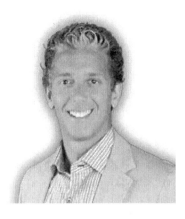

Dr. Rob Kominiarek DO FACOFP
President & Medical Director
Alpha Male Medical Institute

Find Dr. Rob online:

Medical Office:
www.alphamaleinstitute.com

Media Inquiries:
www.americasfitnessdoctor.com

Dr. Rob Kominiarek D.O., FACOFP is a board certified, Fellow of the American College of Osteopathic Family Physicians and a Fellows Crest Award Winner in Family Medicine with advanced training in Age Management Medicine and Hormone Optimization. He is president and medical director of the Alpha Male Medical Institute®. Dr. Rob is a graduate of the Nova-Southeastern University, College of Osteopathic Medicine in Fort Lauderdale, Florida. He completed his residency training at Ohio University, Grandview Hospital and Medical Center in Dayton, Ohio and is an Assistant Clinical Professor at Ohio University. An Amazon Bestselling Author, Dr. Rob is a medical advisor and director to emergency medical services, police departments and radio and television shows across the country. Dr. Rob is a veteran of the United States Army and is a bestselling author with a passion directed towards overall health of the mind and body thru proper nutritional habits, regular exercise, appropriate supplementation, and the intelligent optimization of hormones when clinically indicated. Dr. Rob is an avid athlete who enjoys cycling, swimming, triathlons, soccer, tennis, soaring, skiing Utah, Italian motorcycles, and automobile racing. Dr. Rob is a dedicated father who believes in practicing what he preaches, and as such lives a lifestyle dedicated towards healthy living and regular exercise.

"What are you willing to do that others won't, so your body can perform when theirs cannot?"

APPENDIX

MENU IDEAS

When the meal calls for a piece of fruit, this includes items such as an average-sized apple. When the meal calls for a cup of fruit, it means smaller low glycemic fruits like strawberries, blueberries (LBP's Dr. Rob's little blue powerhouses) or raspberries. Nut butters can be almond, cashew, or peanut.

BREAKFAST

Vanilla Protein Pancakes
1/2cup egg whites
1 whole egg
1/4 of oatmeal
1/4 teaspoon cinnamon
1/4teaspoon vanilla
1 scoop of vanilla protein powder
Cook over low heat with a non-stick spray, use low calorie, and sugar free maple syrup

Chocolate Protein Almond Butter and Banana Pancake
1 egg
1/2 a banana
1/4 of oatmeal
1 teaspoon of almond butter
1 scoop of chocolate protein powder
Cook over low heat with a non-stick spray, use low calorie, sugar free maple syrup

Egg White Scramble Wrap
1 cup of egg whites
1 cup of spinach
1 diced red pepper
1 diced yellow pepper
2 tablespoons of salsa 1 tortilla
Coat a nonstick pan with olive oil spray and over medium heat scramble egg whites then add spinach and peppers. Place in tortilla add salsa and wrap

Egg White Pepper Scramble
2 cups of egg whites
1-1/2 cups of spinach
1 diced red pepper
1 diced yellow pepper
2 tablespoons of salsa
Coat a nonstick pan with olive oil spray and over medium heat scramble egg whites then add spinach and peppers. Top with salsa.

Omelet
1 organic whole egg and 5 whites
Cooked in I tbsp. olive oil, with I oz. cheese and 2 cups spinach, mushrooms, onions mix
1 slice Ezekiel toast with almond butter

Quinoa & rice cereal
½ cup (dry) quinoa and rice
25 g protein powder
1 tsp. Agave nectar
10 walnuts
½ cup of berries

Salmon lox
6 oz. smoked salmon with 1 tbsp. cream cheese and 1 cup fruit or one piece of fruit

Eggs and sausage
1 organic whole egg and 5 whites
4 oz. turkey sausage
1 cup fruit or one piece of fruit

Cinnamon oatmeal & nuts
½ cup (dry) oatmeal
1 scoop protein powder
Cinnamon to taste
10 walnuts or almonds

Ezekiel toast & yogurt
One slice Ezekiel Toast
1 tbsp. nut butter
I cup nonfat Greek yogurt with ½ cup berries

Veggie omelet
 1 cup chopped celery
1/3 cup chopped onions
1/3 cup chopped mushrooms
6 egg whites
½ cup low fat shredded cheese-optional

Bacon Swiss omelet
1 organic whole and 3 egg whites
2 turkey bacon
1oz. shredded Swiss cheese-optional
Cook in 1 tbsp. olive oil or coconut oil
One slice of Ezekiel toast topped with 1 tbsp. natural nut butter

Spinach omelet
1 organic whole egg and 5 egg whites
1 cup each: spinach and mushrooms
1 oz. cheese-optional
Cook with 1 tbsp. olive oil or coconut oil
One slice of Ezekiel toast topped with 1 tbsp. natural nut butter.

Spicy omelet
1 organic whole egg and 2 egg whites
1 small can green chilies
1 oz. Shredded jack cheese-optional
Cook with 1tbsp. Olive oil or coconut oil
One slice ezekiel toast topped with i tbsp. Natural nut butter.

Yogurt parfait
1-cup plain, low- or nonfat greek yogurt
1-cup fresh berries
10 almonds

Eggs and bacon
3 organic egg whites scrambled in 1 tbsp. Olive oil or coconut oil
2-3 strips of turkey bacon

Cheese & fruit
1 cup low fat cottage cheese
I cup fresh berries or 1 small piece of fresh fruit

Omelet with peppers
1 organic whole egg and 4 egg whites
1 cup chopped pepper
2 tbsp. chopped onion
2 tbsp. green salsa
Cook with 1 tbsp. olive oil or coconut oil
One slice of Ezekiel toast topped with 1 tbsp. natural nut butter.

Omelet with broccoli
1 organic whole egg and 2 egg whites
1 cup of ground turkey sausage
1 cup broccoli
Cook with 1tbsp. Olive oil or coconut oil
One slice of ezekiel toast topped with 1 tbsp. Natural nut butter.

Scrambled eggs with cheese
1 organic whole egg and 4 egg whites
1-2 oz. Of your favorite cheese
Cook in 1 tbsp. Olive oil or coconut oil

Greek parfait
1 cup of plain greek yogurt
1 cup fresh mixed berries
10 almonds or walnuts

Oatmeal with protein powder
1 cup steel cut oatmeal
1 scoop chocolate or vanilla whey protein powder
10 walnuts
1 tsp of agave nectar
½ cup of berries

LUNCH & DINNER

Buffalo burger
6-8oz of ground buffalo
Sea salt
Black pepper
Italian seasoning
Red pepper flake
1/2 shallot
1 teaspoon of mustard

Mix all the ingredients in a mixing bowl and form into a pattie and grill

Turkey Burger
6-8oz of ground turkey
Sea salt
Black pepper
Italian seasoning
Red pepper flake
1/2 shallot
1 teaspoon of mustard

Mix all the ingredients in a mixing bowl and form into a pattie and grill

Turkey Chili
1 pound of ground turkey
1 can of tomato sauce
1 can of kidney beans
1 teaspoon of chili powder
Black pepper

Roast turkey
6 oz. Roasted turkey,
I cup steamed broccoli
1 tsp. Apple cider vinegar

Chicken Salad
6oz of chicken
1oz of low fat mayonnaise
1 teaspoon of mustard
1/4 cup of chopped carrots
1/4 cup of chopped celery
1/4 cup of chopped shallots
Black pepper to taste

Filet mignon
Petite filet mignon
6 oz. Sautéed mushrooms
Side salad with apple cider
vinegar

Turkey meatloaf
1 pound of ground turkey
1/2 cup diced shallots
3 chopped garlic cloves, 6 chopped fresh basil leaves
3/4 cup of salsa
Pinch of sea salt & black pepper
1/2 cup of Italian bread crumbs

Pre heat oven to 350 degrees. Mix all the ingredients together in a large bowl, form into a loaf and place into an oven safe dish. Top with more salsa and bake for 30-45 minutes.

Veal Burger
6-8oz of ground veal
Sea salt
Black pepper
Italian seasoning
Red pepper flake
1/2 shallot
1 teaspoon of mustard

Mix all the ingredients in a mixing bowl and form into a pattie and grill.

Crock Pot Salsa Chicken
Place several chicken breasts in a crock-pot
Cover them with your favorite salsa
Turn on low and forget about it
Later in day add your favorite vegetables

I love this one on the weekends for multiple meals and its simplicity

Crab and avocado salad
6 oz. Fresh cooked crab
1 cup chopped celery
Half an haas avocado
Squeezed fresh lemon juice
1 tbsp. Olive oil
1 tsp. Cumin
1 tsp. Turmeric
Mix together and place in an Ezekiel pita

Chicken and vegetables
6 oz. Grilled chicken breast
½ cup of brown rice
2 cups steamed vegetables

Caesar salad with chicken
Large spinach salad 2 tbsp. Caesar dressing
6 oz. Diced, grilled chicken

Tuna Salad
6oz of tuna
1oz of low fat mayonnaise
1/4 cup of chopped carrots
1/4 cup of chopped celery
1/4 cup of chopped shallots
Black pepper to taste

Chicken & lamb kabobs
3 oz. Chicken breast and
3 oz. Lamb
Skewer & grill to desire

Salmon salad
6 oz. Salmon
3oz. Feta cheese
Garden salad mixed vegetables and apple cider vinegar

Chicken or tuna pocket
4-6 oz. Tuna or white meat chicken
1 -2 tbsp. Olive oil mayonnaise
1 cup chopped vegetables
Ezekiel pita

New York strip
6 oz. New York steak
½ sweet potato
Salad with 2 tbsp. Olive oil dressing

Grilled cheese
Ezekiel pita
1 tbsp. Olive oil or coconut oil
1 oz. Cheese your choice
1 large tomato
1 portobello mushroom

Chicken & black beans
½ cup brown rice
½ cup black beans
1 raw onion
1 chicken breast
2 oz. Diced green chilies
7 oz. Diced tomatoes

Grilled fish
4-6 oz. Salmon or white fish
2 cups grilled vegetables
½ cup of brown rice

Turkey burger
4-6 oz. Extra-lean ground turkey breast
I slice cheese-optional
Tomato, onion, salsa
Ezekiel bun

Broiled tilapia
4-6 oz. Broiled tilapia
1 cup steamed asparagus
½ cup brown rice

Beef stew
6 oz. Lean beef
1 cup lentils
1 cup each celery, carrots, onions, cabbage, spinach, and sweet potato

Stir fry
6 oz. Chicken, shrimp or scallops stir-fried in 2 tbsp. Olive oil or coconut oil with 2 cups mixed vegetables
1/2 cup brown rice

London broil
6 oz. London broil
2 cup sautéed green beans
½ sweet potato

Roasted chicken
6 oz. Roasted chicken breast
2 cups of broccoli
½ cup of black beans with salsa

Chicken cobb salad
6 oz. Fresh greens
6 oz. Grilled chicken
1 hard-boiled egg
Fresh chopped tomato
1/2 cup black olives
1/2 avocado
2 oz. Apple cider vinegar dressing

Roasted turkey
6 oz. Roasted turkey
1/2 sweet potato
2 cups steamed broccoli

Roasted chicken & steamed vegetables
6 oz. Roasted seasoned chicken breast.
2 cups steamed vegetables

Roasted lamb
6 oz. Roasted lamb
10 asparagus spears
1 cup mushrooms sautéed in olive oil
½ sweet potato

Tuna salad with bibb lettuce
Can of tuna topped on a bed of bibb lettuce
Chopped cucumbers, tomatoes, onions
Drizzle with olive oil vinaigrette dressing

Salmon salad
6 oz. Salmon on
2 cups fresh greens.
1 cup celery, onions, mushrooms
Red wine vinaigrette dressing and fresh-squeezed lemon juice

Grilled chicken kabobs
6 oz. Chicken marinated in teriyaki
1-cup fresh cubed pineapple
1 green bell pepper cut into squares

GLUTEN-FREE FOODS

Spinach omelet
1 organic egg and 5 whites
Scrambled in 1 tbsp. Olive oil or
coconut oil with 1-cup spinach and
2 tbsp. Feta cheese

Breakfast chicken
6 oz. Grilled chicken
1 cup black beans
1 tbsp. Salsa
½ quinoa

Veggie omelet
6 egg whites
1 cup chopped onions, celery,
mushrooms
6 egg whites
1/2 cup low fat shredded cheese
optional

Yogurt parfait
1-cup low fat yogurt
1 cup berries or chopped fruit
10 walnuts

GLUTEN FREE LUNCH AND DINNER

Beef lentil soup
10 oz. Beef soup with lentils, celery,
onions, carrots, sweet potato, and
mushrooms

Chicken & vegetables
6 oz. Grilled chicken breast
½ sweet potato
2 cup steamed broccoli

Pick your protein salad
6 oz. Tuna, salmon, sardine, chicken
Bibb lettuce with chopped
vegetables
10 chopped walnuts
Apple cider vinegar dressing

Shrimp salad
6 oz. Giant shrimp
Bibb lettuce
½ avocado
2 tbsp. Green salsa
1 cup black beans

Turkey/bison burger
6 oz. Ground turkey or bison
Ezekiel bun with tomato
2 cup steamed vegetables

Roasted lamb
40-oz. Bone-in roasted lamb chops
2 cup steamed vegetable

Grilled salmon
6 oz. Grilled salmon
2 cup grilled vegetables
2 cups butternut squash

Broiled fish
6 oz. Broiled tilapia
2 cup steamed broccoli
½ sweet potato

Skirt steak
6 oz. Skirt Steak
½ sweet potato
2 cups mixed vegetables

Filet mignon
8 oz. Filet mignon
10 asparagus spears
½ brown rice

INCIDENTALS

Vanilla Protein Pudding
6 scoops of vanilla protein powder
1-1/2 cups of water
Blend with a mixer to desired consistency and top with crushed almonds and cinnamon

Chocolate Protein Pudding
6 scoops of chocolate protein powder
1-1/2 cups of water
Blend with a mixer to desired consistency and top with crushed walnuts

Basil Pesto
1cup extra virgin olive oil
1 stuffed cup of fresh basil
Pinch of sea salt & black pepper
3-garlic cloves
Teaspoon of pine nuts
1/2 cup of grated Parmesan cheese
Place all the ingredients in a food processor and blend until processed

Fennel Pesto
1cup extra virgin olive oil
1 chopped fresh fennel bulb
Pinch of sea salt & black pepper
3 garlic cloves

Place olive oil in a skillet and warm over medium heat. Caramelize the chopped fresh fennel with the garlic and add a pinch of sea salt and black pepper. Place the mixture in a bowl.

Butter Nut Squash

Peal a Butter Nut Squash, cut in half and remove the seeds. Dice into half inch cubes, place on a baking sheet covered with aluminum foil. Spray with extra virgin olive oil, sprinkle with sea salt and cinnamon. Broil on high for 20 min, and remove.

Southwest Quinoa Salad

1 cup of quinoa
1 clove of garlic
1 red pepper
1 yellow pepper
1 onion
¼ cup of cilantro
2 tablespoons of olive oil

Bring water to a boil and add quinoa, return to a boil then simmer till done and cover. Placed quinoa in a large mixing bowl and add chopped ingredients, olive oil and mix together.

Dr. Rob's salad dressing

1 cup of extra virgin olive oil
1 minced garlic clove
Italian seasoning
1 tablespoon of lemon juice

Whisk ingredients together in a small bowl. 1 teaspoon is about 60 calories.

PROTEIN SHAKES

The below protein shakes are my preferences. Feel free to use whichever flavor you like and the fruits you prefer. You can use water, skim milk, or almond milk in any recipe. *Mix in blender to desired consistency.*

Peach & yogurt shake
8 oz. Water
1 organic peach
2 tbsp. Low fat yogurt
1 scoop vanilla protein powder

Banana nut chocolate
8 oz. Unsweetened almond milk
1 small banana
1 tbsp. Peanut butter
1 scoop chocolate protein powder

Blueberries & yogurt shake
8 oz. Water
1-cup organic blueberries
2 tbsp. Low fat yogurt
1 scoop vanilla protein powder

Chocolate & almonds
8 oz. Water
2 tbsp. Almond butter
1 tbsp. Plain yogurt
1 scoop chocolate protein powder

Espresso shake
1 shot espresso
8 oz. Water
3-4 ice cubes
1 scoop cookies and cream protein powder

Orange shake
8 oz. Water
1 peeled orange
1 scoop vanilla protein powder

Chocolate cake shake
8 oz. Water
1 tbsp. Half and half cream
1 tbsp. Cream of coconut
1 scoop chocolate protein powder

Chocolate peanut butter
8 oz. Water
10 walnuts
1 tbsp. Peanut butter
1 scoop chocolate protein powder

Apple shake with pecans
8 oz. Water
1 small organic apple
1 tsp. Cinnamon
1 tsp. Nutmeg
1 oz. Pecans
1 scoop vanilla protein powder

Green lantern shake
1 cup of water, 2-3 ice cubes
1 scoop of vanilla protein powder
¼ tsp. Of cinnamon
1-cup baby spinach
1 celery stalk
4 slices of seedless cucumber
½ of an organic green apple

MACRONUTRIENTS: THE FUEL FOR YOUR NEW BODY

The following lists are some of the macronutrients you read about in chapter 9. While these lists may seem small, keep this in mind. The overwhelming majority of people eat the same SEVEN foods their entire life. Subconsciously you choose the foods you like to eat because of a certain taste profile. These lists are not all inclusive and you may choose to add any item you like. But first, know where that item belongs in the macronutrient profile. Is it a protein, a vegetable carbohydrate, fruit carbohydrate, starchy carbohydrate or a fat. That being said, I highly recommend that you only use the starchy carbohydrates and healthy fats I have suggested in the lists below when you make your meals.

PROTEINS (each serving approximately 200 calories)

- Chicken 6oz
- Salmon 6oz
- Tuna 6oz
- Sardines 6oz
- Red meat (fillet) 6oz
- Egg whites 1 3/4 cup
- Protein powder (refer to product label for calorie per serving)

- Turkey 6oz
- Turkey bacon 4 slices
- Protein pancakes
- Protein pudding

FATS

- Extra virgin olive oil (1 teaspoon approximately 60 calories)
- Dr. Rob's salad dressing (1 teaspoon approximately 60 calories)
- Dr. Rob's fennel pesto (1 teaspoon approximately 60 calories)
- Dr. Rob's basil pesto (1 teaspoon approximately 60 calories)
- Avocado (one tablespoon approximately 120 calories)
- Almonds (one oz. approximately 200 calories)
- Walnuts (one oz. approximately 200 calories)
- Pistachios (one oz. approximately 200 calories)
- Almond butter (1 tablespoon approximately 90 calories)

CARBOHYDRATES

STARCHY CARBOHYDRATES (each serving approximately 200 calories)
*Starchy carbohydrates have a red light because they raise your blood sugar levels.

- Black beans 1 cup
- Pinto beans 1 cup
- Lentils 1 cup
- Hummus 1 cup
- Oatmeal 1 cup
- Pasta 1 cup
- Quinoa 1 cup Rice 1 cup
- Sweet potato 1 average size
- Squash 4 cups
- Carrots 4 cups
- Flourless sprout grain bread 2 slices (160 calories)
- 1 Whole-wheat tortilla (80 calories)

FRUIT CARBOHYDRATES (each serving approximately 100 calories) *Fruit carbohydrates have a yellow light because they raise your blood sugar levels.

- Apple 1 average size
- Banana 1 average size
- Peach 1 average size
- Pear 1 average size
- Orange 1 average size
- Grapefruit 1 average size
- Figs dried 1/4 cup
- Grapes 1 cup
- Blueberries 1 cup
- Strawberries 2 cups

VEGETABLE CARBOHYDRATE (each serving cooked 1 cup approximately 50 calories)

- Broccoli
- Broccoli Rabe
- Asparagus
- Cauliflower
- Mushrooms
- Peas
- Peppers
- String beans
- Zucchini
- Artichoke

* The preferred methods for preparation of foods are to grill, bake, broil your protein sources; steam, grill, broil your vegetables and fruits and leafy greens consume in their natural state.

* Note well. It is in your best health interest that you try to consume as many of these above food items in organic, free range, grass-fed, cage free, no pesticides, no herbicides, no hormones or antibiotics as possible The following uncooked leafy greens are 2 cups approximately 50 calories.

- Spinach (Baby)
- Spinach
- Arugula
- Herb salad mix
- Romaine salad
- European salad mix
- Swiss chard

These carbohydrate tables on the following pages give the GI and GL values for common foods so that you can see which ones are best to add to your meals. Any food with an asterisk has a GI/GL equal to zero. The lower the number the slower it will raise your blood sugar.

FOOD	GI	GL
Agave Nectar	19	1
Alfalfa Sprouts	*	*
Apple	38	6
Artichokes	*	*
Asparagus	*	*
Black Beans	30	5
Broccoli, Cauliflower	*	*
Brussels Sprouts	*	*
Cabbage	*	*
Carrots	41	2
Celery	*	*
Cucumber, Zucchini	*	*
Eggplant	*	*
Grapefruit	25	3
Green Beans	*	*
Green Peas	51	4
Garlic & Ginger	*	*
Honey	35	6
Hummus	6	1
Lemon, Lime	*	*
Lettuce	*	*
Mushrooms	*	*
Orange	42	5
Peach	42	5
Pear	38	4
Raspberries	40	1
Cherries	22	3
Spinach	*	*
Squash	*	*
Strawberries	40	1
Sweet Potato	44	11
Tomato	38	1

FOOD	GI	GL
9 Grain Multi Grain Bread	43	6
100% Stone-ground Wheat	59	7
All Bran Cereal	34	5
Apricots	57	7
Apricots	30	9
Banana	52	13
Beets	64	5
Bran Muffin	28	3
Brown Rice	50	24
Cantaloupe	67	4
Chapatti	27	6
Tortellini	50	10
Grapes	53	8
Kiwi	53	6
Mango	51	8
Muesli	40	8
Oat Bran and Honey Bread	45	7
Oat Bran	55	3
Oatmeal	52	11
Papaya	56	5
Pita Bread	57	10
Polenta	68	9
Potatoes	72	16
Pumpernickel Bread	50	5
Quinoa	51	9
Rye Bread	51	7
Semolina	55	6
Sourdough Wheat Bread	54	8
Spaghetti	27	14
Watermelon	76	4
Wild rice	57	18

FOOD	GI	GL
Blueberry Muffin	59	17
Candy Bar	62	25
Chocolate Cake	38	20
Corn Flakes	77	20
Corn Pops Cereal	80	21
Couscous	65	21
Croissant	67	17
Cupcake	73	19
Dates	45	18
Fettuccini	40	18
French Fries	75	22
Graham Crackers	77	14
Ice Cream	37	31
Instant Noodles	67	34
Jasmine White Rice	89	46
Macaroni	47	23
Maple Syrup	54	10
Marshmallows	62	12
Millet	71	25
Pancakes	67	15
Pop-Tarts	70	25
Processed Fruit Snack	99	24
Raisins	64	28
Rice Cakes	82	17
Risotto	69	29
Skittles	70	32
Stuffing	74	16
White Bagel	72	25

DAIRY	SERVING SIZE	PROTEIN (g)
Cottage Cheese	1 cup	15
Egg Whites	Six large	24
Plain Greek Yogurt (2% fat or less)	8oz.	16
Omega-3 Egg (with yolk)	One large	6.3

FISH & SEAFOOD	SERVING SIZE	PROTEIN (g)
Lobster Meat	5 oz.	24
Lump Crab Meat	5 oz.	22
Mahi Mahi	5 oz.	26.9
Red Snapper	5 oz.	32
Sea Bass	5 oz.	27
Shrimp	5 oz.	24
Swordfish	5 oz.	29
Canned Tuna	5 oz.	39
Wild Salmon Fillet	5 oz.	35
Tuna	5 oz.	34
POULTRY	SERVING SIZE	PROTEIN (g)
Chicken	5 oz.	30
Turkey	5 oz.	32

MEAT	SERVING SIZE	PROTEIN (g)
Pork Chop	5 oz.	25
Grass-fed Beef	5 oz.	27
Lamb	5 oz.	30
Beef (lean cuts)	5 oz.	35

GROCERYLIST

VEGETABLES	FRUITS
Asparagus	Apples
Broccoli Spinach	Avocados
Cabbage	Bananas
Carrots	Berries
Cauliflower	Grapefruit
Celery	Grapes
Collard Greens	Nectarines
Eggplant	Oranges
Garlic	Pears
Green Beans	Plums
Lettuce	Tomatoes
Mushrooms	Peaches
Olives	Blueberries
Onions	Strawberries
Peppers	Raspberries
Radishes	
Edamame	
Water Chestnuts	
Yams or Sweet Potatoes	
DAIRY	**SEAFOOD**
Cheese	Mackerel
Cottage Cheese (low-fat)	Salmon
Egg Beaters	Sardines
Eggs (organic, free range)	Shrimp
Milk (1% or skim)	Steel Head Trout
Plain Yogurt	Swordfish
	Tuna
	Halibut
	Tilapia
	Orange Roughy
	Scallops

MEAT & POULTRY	
Beef	
Chicken Breasts	
Pork	
Turkey Breasts or Lean Ground Turkey	
ADDITIONAL ITEMS	
Steel cut Oatmeal	
Agave Nectar light	Extra virgin Olive Oil
Brown or Wild Rice	Protein Powder (Beverly International)
Mayonnaise *(olive oil based)*	Spices
Mustard	Stevia
Natural Peanut Butter	Tea
Raw Nuts	Vinaigrette Dressing

RECOMMENDED READING

If you are interested in learning more about men's health and wellness, I recommend reading the following publications.

"Keep It Up" The Power of Precision Medicine to Conquer Low T and Revitalize Your Life by Florence Comite, M.D.

"Mastering the Life Plan" The Essential Steps to Achieving Great Health and a Leaner, Stronger, and Sexier Body by Jeffry S. Life, M.D. Ph.D.

"Reverse Heart Disease Now" Stop Deadly Cardiovascular Plaque Before It's Too Late by Drs. Stephen T. Sinatra, M.D. & James C. Roberts, M.D.

"Testosterone for Life" Recharge Your Vitality, Sex Drive, Muscle Mass & Overall Health by Dr. Abraham Morgentaler, M.D.

"The Blood Sugar Solution" The UltraHealthy Program for Losing Weight, Preventing Disease, and Feeling Great Now! By Dr. Mark Hyman, M.D.

"The Disease Delusion" Conquering the Causes of Chronic Illness for a Healthier, Longer, and Happier Life by Dr. Jeffrey S. Bland

"The Life Plan" How Any Man Can Achieve Lasting Health, Great Sex, and a Stronger, Leaner Body by Jeffry S. Life, M.D. Ph.D.

"The Testosterone Syndrome" The Critical Factor for Energy, Health, & Sexuality – Reversing the Male Menopause by Dr. Eugene Shippen, M.D.

REFERENCES

Geta S. et. Al. In vitro and invivo impairment of alpha 2 adrenergic receptor dependent antilipolysis by fatty acids in human adipose tissue Horm Metab Res. (2001).

Ardioluze JL et. Al. Subcutaneous tissue blood flow varies between superior and inferior levels of the anterior abdominal wall Int J Obesity (2004).

Arner P et. Al. Adrenergic regulation of lipolysis in site at rest and during exercise. J Clin Invest (1990).

Chritmass MA et. al. Effect of Work and recovery duration on skeletal muscle oxygenation and fuel use during sustained intermittent exercise. Eur J Appl Physiol (1999).

Glueck, CJ., Wang, P. Testosterone therapy, thrombosis, thrombophilia, cardiovascular events. Metabolism (2014).

Haring R, Ittermann T, Völzke H, Krebs A, Zygmunt M, Felix SB, Grabe HJ, Nauck M, Wallaschofski H. "Prevalence, incidence and risk factors of testosterone deficiency in a population-based cohort of men: results from the study of health in Pomerania." Aging Male. 2010 Dec; 13(4): 247-57. doi: 10.3109/13685538.2010.487553. Epub 2010 May 26.

Power ML and J Shulkin. Sex differences in fat storage, fat metabolism and health risks from obesity, possible evolutionary origins. Br J Nutr (2007). Hämäläinen E, Adlercreutz H, Puska P, Pietinen P. "Diet and serum sex hormones in healthy men." J Steroid Biochem. 1984 Jan; 20(1): 459-64.

Pilz S1, Frisch S, Koertke H, Kuhn J, Dreier J, Obermayer-Pietsch B, Wehr E, Zittermann A. "Effect of vitamin D supplementation on testosterone levels in men." Horm Metab Res. 2011 Mar;43(3):223-5. doi: 10.1055/s-0030-1269854. Epub 2010 Dec 10.

Doucet E. et al. Reduction of visceral adipose tissue during weight loss. Eur J Clin Nutr (2002).

Netter A. Hartoma R.,Nahoul K., Effect of zinc administration on plasma testosterone, dihydrotestosterone, and sperm count. Arch Androl 1981 Aug;7(1):69-73.

Ahtiainen JP, Hulmi JJ, Kraemer WJ, Lehti M, Nyman K, Selänne H, Alen M, Pakarinen A, Komulainen J, Kovanen V, Mero AA, Häkkinen K, "Heavy resistance exercise training and skeletal muscle androgen receptor expression in younger and older men." Steroids. 2011; 76(1-2):183-92

McArdle W.D. and F. Katch V., L. Katch. Exercise Physiology: Energy, Nutrition, and Human Performance. Philadelphia: Lippincott Williams & Wilkins, (2007).

Rahimi R1, Qaderi M, Faraji H, Boroujerdi SS. "Effects of very short rest periods on hormonal responses to resistance exercise in men". J Strength Cond Res. 2010 Jul; 24(7): 1851-9. doi: 10.1519/JSC.0b013e3181ddb265.

Smith A, Toone R, Peacock O, Drawer S, Stokes K, Cook C. "Dihydrotestosterone is elevated following sprint exercise in healthy young men." J Appl Physiol 1985. 2013; 114(10): 1435-40.

Mehta, Josephs RA, Testosterone and cortisol jointly regulate dominance: evidence for a dual-hormone hypothesis. Horm Behav. 2010 Nov; 58(5): 898-906. doi: 10.1016/j.yhbeh.2010.08.020. Epub 2010 Sep 15.

Azevedo FR1, Ikeoka D, Caramelli B. Effects of intermittent fasting on metabolism in men. Rev Assoc Med Bras. 2013 Mar-Apr; 59(2): 167-73. doi: 10.1016/j.ramb.2012.09.003.

Ridker, PM, A Pradhan, JG MacFaadyen, P Libby, RJ Glynn. "Cardiovascular benefits and diabetes risks of statin therapy in primary prevention: An analysis from the JUPITER trial." Lancet (2012) 565-71.

Price M and Moss P. The effects of work:rest duration on physiology and perceptual responses during intermittent exercise and performance. J Sports Science (2007).

Horowitz JF. Fatty acid mobilization from adipose tissue during exercise. Trends Endocr Metab. (2003).

Key TJ, Roe L, Thorogood M, Moore JW, Clark GM, Wang DY. "Testosterone, sex hormone-binding globulin, calculated free testosterone, and oestradiol in male vegans and omnivores." Br J Nutr. 1990; 64(1): 111-9.

YU, G, and AM Traish. "Induced testosterone deficiency: From clinical presentation of fatigue, erectile dysfunction, and muscle atrophy to insulin resistance and diabetes." Hormone Molecular Biology and Clinical Investigation (2011).

Ecotoxicol Environ Saf. 2013 May;91:129-38. doi: 10.1016/j.ecoenv.2013.01.022. Epub 2013 Mar 7.

Basaria, S, AD Coviello, TG Travison, TW Storer, WR Farwell, AM Jette, R Eder, "Adverse events associated with testosterone administration." New England Journal of Medicine 363.2 (2010) 109-22

J Strength Cond Res. 2010 Apr;24(4):1125-30. doi: 10.1519/JSC.0b013e3181c7c655.

Environ Health Perspect. 2011 Jul;119(7):989-96. doi: 10.1289/ehp.1003220. Epub 2011 Feb 24.

Most plastic products release estrogenic chemicals: a potential health problem that can be solved. Yang CZ, Yaniger SI, Jordan VC, Klein DJ, Bittner GD.

Metabolism. 2014 Aug;63(8):989-994. doi: 10.1016/j.metabol.2014.05.005. Epub 2014 May 15. Testosterone therapy, thrombosis, thrombophilia, cardiovascular events. Glueck CJ1, Wang P2.

(Zhang Y et al. A Strategy for Cancer Prevention: Stimulation of the Nrf2-ARE signaling pathway. Mol Cancer Therapy 2004;3(7) July

Marks, LS, DL Hess, FJ Dorsey, M Luz Macarian, PB Cruz Santos, and VE Tyler. "Tissue effects of saw palmetto and finasteride: Use of biopsy core for in situ quantification of prostatic androgen." Urology 57.5 (2001): 999-1005.

Rhoden, EL and A Morgentaler, "Risk of testosterone replacement therapy and recommendations for monitoring." New England Journal of Medicine 350 (2005): 482-92.

Murphy, A "Vitamin D Levels Linked to Prostate Cancer Risk" Clinical Cancer Research, 2014, May 1;20: 2289-99

American Journal of Clinical Nutrition, 2014, May; 99(5) 1015-25, "Correcting Low Vitamin D Results in Weight Loss and Reduced Inflammation".

Mueller M, van den Beld AW, Bots ML, Grobbee DE, Lamberts SW van der Schouw YT. "Endogenous sex Hormones and Progression of Carotid Atherosclerosis in the Elderly". Circulation. 2004 May 4;109:2074-9

Stattin P, Lumme S, Tenkanen L, et al. "High Levels of Circulating Testosterone are not Associated with Increased Prostate Cancer Risk." Int J Cancer. 2004 Jan; 108: 418-24

Svartberg J, Jenssen T, Sundsfjord J, Jorde R. "The Association of Endogenous Testosterone and Sex Hormone Binding Globulin with Glcosylated Hemoglobin Levels, in Community Dwelling Men. The Tromso Study. Diabetes Metabolism. 2004 Feb; 30, 29-34

Glueck CJ, Richardson-Royer C, Schultz R, Burger T, Bowe D, Padda J, et al. Testosterone therapy, thrombophilia-hypofi- brinolysis, and hospitalization for deep venous thrombosis- pulmonary embolus: an exploratory, hypothesis-generating study. Clin Appl Thromb Hemost 2014;20:244–9.

Glueck CJ, Bowe D, Valdez A, Wang P. Thrombosis in three postmenopausal women receiving testosterone therapy for low libido. Womens Health (Lond Engl) 2013;9:405–10.

Glueck CJ, Goldenberg N, Budhani S, Lotner D, Abuchaibe C, Gowda M, et al. Thrombotic events after starting exogenous testosterone in men with previously undiagnosed familial thrombophilia. Transl Res 2011;158:225–34.

Glueck Charles J, Friedman J, Hafeez A, Hassan A, Wang P. Testosterone, thrombophilia, thrombosis. Blood Coagul Fi- brinolysis 2014 [epub 2014]. Glueck CJ, Richardson-Royer C, Schultz R, Burger T, Labitue F, Riaz MK, et al. Testosterone, thrombophilia, and thrombosis. Clin Appl Thromb Hemost 2014;20:22–30.

Pandit RS, Glueck CJ. Testosterone, anastrozole, factor V Leiden heterozygosity and osteonecrosis of the jaws. Blood Coagul Fibrinolysis 2014;25:286–8.

Spitzer M, Huang G, Basaria S, Travison TG, Bhasin S. Risks and benefits of testosterone therapy in older men. Nat Rev Endocrinol 2013;9:414–24.

Marchioli R, Finazzi G, Specchia G, Cacciola R, Cavazzina R, Cilloni D, et al. Cardiovascular events and intensity of treatment in polycythemia vera. N Engl J Med 2013;368:22–33.

Xu L, Freeman G, Cowling BJ, Schooling CM. Testosterone therapy and cardiovascular events among men: a systematic review and meta-analysis of placebo-controlled randomized trials. BMC Med 2013;11:108:1–12.

Fernandez-Balsells MM, Murad MH, Lane M, Lampropulos JF, Albuquerque F, Mullan RJ, et al. Clinical review 1: Adverse effects of testosterone therapy in adult men: a systematic review and meta-analysis. J Clin Endocrinol Metab 2010;95:2560–75.

Baskurt OK, Meiselman HJ. Iatrogenic hyperviscosity and thrombosis. Semin Thromb Hemost 2012;38:854–64.

Peerschke EI, Silver RT, Weksler BB, Yin W, Bernhardt B, Varon D. Examination of platelet function in whole blood under dynamic flow conditions with the cone and plate(let) analyzer: effect of erythrocytosis and thrombocytosis. Am J Clin Pathol 2007;127:422–8.

Ajayi AA, Mathur R, Halushka PV. Testosterone increases human platelet thromboxane A2 receptor density and aggregation responses. Circulation 1995;91:2742–7.

Stapleton PA, James ME, Goodwill AG, Frisbee JC. Obesity and vascular dysfunction. Pathophysiology 2008;15:79–89.

Death AK, McGrath KC, Sader MA, Nakhla S, Jessup W, Handelsman DJ, et al. Dihydrotestosterone promotes vascular cell adhesion molecule-1 expression in male human endothelial cells via a nuclear factor-kappaB-dependent pathway. Endocrinology 2004;145:1889–97.

Lycette JL, Luoh SW, Beer TM, Deloughery TG. Acute bilateral pulmonary emboli occurring while on adjuvant aromatase inhibitor therapy with anastrozole: case report and review of the literature. Breast Cancer Res Treat 2006;99:249–55.

Svartberg J, Braekkan SK, Laughlin GA, Hansen JB. Endogenous sex hormone levels in men are not associated with risk of venous thromboembolism: the Tromso study. Eur J Endocrinol 2009;160:833–8.

Pamukcu B, Lip GY, Devitt A, Griffiths H, Shantsila E. The role of monocytes in atherosclerotic coronary artery disease. Ann Med 2010;42:394–403.

Urhausen A, Torsten A, Wilfried K. Reversibility of the effects on blood cells, lipids, liver function and hormones in former anabolic-androgenic steroid abusers. J Steroid Biochem Mol Biol 2003;84:369–75.

Swerdloff RS, Wang C, Cunningham G, Dobs A, Iranmanesh A, Matsumoto AM, et al. Long-term pharmacokinetics of trans- dermal testosterone gel in hypogonadal men. J Clin Endocri- nol Metab 2000;85:4500–10.

Hoibraaten E, Qvigstad E, Andersen TO, Mowinckel MC, Sandset PM. The effects of hormone replacement therapy (HRT) on hemostatic variables in women with previous venous thromboembolism – results from a randomized, double-blind, clinical trial. Thromb Haemost 2001;85:775–81.

Hulley S, Grady D, Bush T, Furberg C, Herrington D, Riggs B, et al. Randomized trial of estrogen plus progestin for secondary prevention of coronary heart disease in postmenopausal women. Heart and Estrogen/progestin Replacement Study (HERS) Research Group. JAMA 1998;280:605–13.

Copyright and Trademark Notices

Limits of Liability & Disclaimers of Warranties

This book/eBook is a general educational health related information product.

As an express condition to reading this book/eBook, you understand and agree to the following terms:

This book's/eBook's content is not a substitute for direct, personal, professional medical care and diagnosis. None of the exercises or treatments, including products or services mentioned in this book/eBook should be performed or otherwise used without the clearance from your physician or health care provider.

There may be risks associated with participating in activities or using products mentioned in this book/eBook for people in poor health or with pre-existing physical or mental conditions.

Because these risks exist, you will not use such products or participate in such activities if you are in poor health or have pre-existing mental or physical condition. If you choose to participate in these risks, you do so of your own free will and accord, knowingly and voluntarily assuming all risks associated with such activities.

The materials in this book/eBook are provided "as is" and without warranties of any kind either expressed or implied.

The Author disclaims all warranties, expressed or implied, including, but not limited to, implied warranties of merchantability and fitness for a particular purpose. The Author does not warrant that defects will be corrected, or that the site or the server that makes this book/eBook available is free of viruses or other harmful components. The Author does not warrant or make any representations regarding the use or the results of the use of the materials in this book/eBook in terms of their correctness, accuracy, reliability, or otherwise. Applicable law may not allow the exclusion of implied warranties, so the above exclusion may not apply to you.

Under no circumstances, including, but not limited to, negligence, shall the Author be liable for any special or consequential damages that result from the use of, or the inability to use this book/eBook, even if the Author or his authorized representative has been advised of the possibility of such damages. Applicable law may not allow the limitation or exclusion of liability or incidental or consequential damages, so the above limitation or exclusion may not apply to you. In no event shall the Author's total liability to you for all damages, losses, and causes of action (weather in contract, tort, including but not limited to, negligence or otherwise) exceed the amount paid by you, if any, for this book/eBook.

You agree to hold the Author of this book/eBook, the Author's owners, agents, affiliates, and employees harmless from any and all liability for all claims for damages due to injuries, including attorney fees and costs, incurred by you or caused to third parties by you, arising out of the products, services, and activities discussed in this book/eBook, excepting only claims for gross negligence or intentional tort.

You agree that any and all claims for gross negligence or intentional tort shall be settled solely by confidential binding arbitration per the American Arbitration Association's commercial arbitration rules. All arbitration must occur in the municipality where the Author's principal place of business is located.

Arbitration fees and costs shall be split equally, and you are solely responsible for your own lawyer fees.

Facts and information are believed to be accurate at the time they were placed in this book/eBook. All data provided in this book/eBook is to be used for information purpose only. The information contained within is not intended to provide specific physical or mental health advice, or any other advice whatsoever, for any individual or company and should not be relied upon in that regard. The services described are only offered in jurisdictions where they may be legally offered. Information provided is not all-inclusive, and is limited to information that is made available and such information should not be relied upon as all-inclusive or accurate.

For more information about this policy please contact the Author at the email address listed in the Copyright notice for this book/eBook.

IF YOU DO NOT AGREE WITH THESE TERMS AND EXPRESS CONDITIONS, DO NOT READ THIS BOOK/EBOOK. YOUR USE OF THIS BOOK/EBOOK, PRODUCTS, SERVICES, AND ANY PARTICIPATION IN ACTIVITIES MENTIONED ON THIS BOOK/EBOOK, MEAN THAT YOU ARE AGREEING TO BE LEGALLY BOUND BY THESE TERMS.

Made in the USA
Lexington, KY
17 July 2016